Seldom does a person come along who can simply and easily express the essence of health and well-being as Dr. Greg Venning.

In his book Thrive *he takes you on a logical journey through what it is to be healthy. This is not another fad, new age health rant. There are no expensive foods, gizmos or gadgets to buy. There is just solid common sense application of scientifically validated and substantiated facts.*

Dr. Venning elegantly covers the four truths of a vitalistic lifestyle and how to embrace them in order to live a bigger life.

You will learn more about the delicate ecosystem that your body is and how you are one with nature. As you gain this awareness you will trust in your innate intelligence and the vitality that springs from inside out.

If you are looking for a way to make your mind, body and world a better place to inhabit then this book is for you.

Dr. Mark Postles
Speaker, professional development expert, chiropractor and author.
Board Member of the New Zealand College of Chiropractic
Board Member of the Spinal Research Foundation

***

It's so accessible and easy to read.
Andrew Baxter, Head of Business Development, WWF

***

WHAT PEOPLE ARE SAYING ABOUT THRIVE!

It's unlike any other book on health I've ever read.

Liezl van Wyk, Director Design Line Architects & Interiors

***

This book is for anyone who's fed-up with being manipulated by conventional SICKCARE professionals; who know that they can be healthier than they are; who want unlimited health and wellness. THRIVE! will change your life and any preconceived notions you may hold about your health and vitality.

Robin Stuart-Clark – Publishing Print Matters (Pty) Ltd.

***

Dr Venning makes me want to be a better man and Thrive! gives me the tools to get it done.

Dr Adam L. Smith
B.Chiro.Sc, M.Chiro (Macq), RPS Cert (NHS - UK)
Chiropractor
Board Secretary Chiropractors' Association of Australia (QLD)
Product Evaluation Committee Member CAA National
Chiropractic Program Reference Committee Central Queensland University

***

This book is for anyone that wants a longer and healthier life. Living in a world where sedentary living is getting more frequent, food is getting worse, and all types of stress are affecting us in a greater way, this book gives us hope in a period of darkness.

Jaime Pinillos Montaño, D.C. ACP
Chiropractor
IFCO Student Global Representative
BCC Philosophy Instructor

***

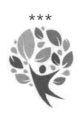

THRIVE!

Only for those who want to be healthy

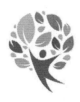

DR GREG VENNING
WITH ELAN LOHMANN

ABOUT THE AUTHOR – DR GREG VENNING

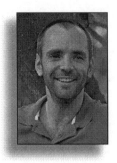 DR GREG VENNING is a husband, a father, developer of Upgrade Your Life, founder of Peak Chiropractic and recipient of the Chiropractic Association of South Africa's Excellence Award. In demand as a Chiropractor, hard-hitting speaker and coach, Greg has helped people of all ages to improve their levels of well-being and lead richer lives.

Greg is not like other doctors; he is interested in creating health, not treating disease. From babies and children to full time mums and from office athletes to elite sportsmen, Greg has helped them all reach greater levels of well-being. He has worked with national sports teams and some of South Africa's biggest companies.

As a Certified Wellness Professional, Greg is well versed in the science of wellness and what our minds and bodies need through nutrition, movement and headspace to create health. He's a nerd at heart and never stops learning about new ways to help you feel and function better so that you can live a fuller life.

It was his own health challenges that led him to search for better ways of looking after people and now Dr Greg applies these principles with everyone he serves.

Human potential and personal performance are Dr Greg's driving passions and he believes you were born to be brilliant. By reconnecting with your in-born potential you can transform your life.

www.thrivelifestyle.solutions
www.capetownchiro.com
@DrGregVenning

AUTHOR'S NOTE

TO HONOUR THE PRIVACY of the people I work with, in telling their stories I have changed their names and all personal details that might identify them. At times I have combined the experiences of two or more similar people into a single story but all of the elements of the stories are factual.

The purpose of this book is to complement, amplify and supplement other texts. You are urged to read all available material, learn as much as possible about health and well-being and tailor the information to your individual needs.

The information contained in this book is for education purposes only, it cannot replace advice or diagnosis by a qualified health care practitioner. If you have symptoms, including but not limited to any that resemble symptoms described in this book, then you should visit your holistically-oriented health care practitioner.

Neither the publisher nor the author shall be liable or responsible for any loss or damage allegedly arising from any information or suggestion in this book.

ABOUT THE AUTHOR – ELAN LOHMANN

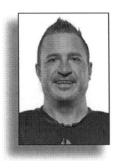 AFTER 12 YEARS in the online media industry in various top management positions, Elan Lohmann successfully reached Executive-level in a listed company by age 34 – including powerful positions such as the General Manager of News24 and the Group Head of Times Media's digital division. Although he was regarded as someone who handled pressure well, it took its toll on him: Elan experienced depression, was under huge stress and hardly slept.

Until February 2012, Elan was an overweight chain smoker propelled by adrenalin and propped up by caffeine and nicotine. Inactive and on the couch living an ultra-unhealthy lifestyle for the majority of his adult life he decided to turn back the clock and begin to thrive with a life of healthier choices.

In September 2012 he simply walked away from a career with a handsome salary. Using his savings he bravely entered into a world of uncertainty as an entrepreneur to pursue a simpler, healthier lifestyle and a new purpose in life: to help others live an optimised life. Many of his industry colleagues thought he was mad. But he had a dream and set himself a vision of inspiring 100,000 South Africans to live a healthier lifestyle.

Elan began with a mere 600 members in his community, many of whom were simply friends and friends of friends, but good news spreads. Cape Town-based, Elan is the founder and fearless leader of Sleekgeek, a South African support group of over 50 000 people – and growing – united by the desire to practise a healthy lifestyle.

The Sleekgeek Code of Conduct is: Respect, Uplift and Inspire.

www.Sleekgeek.co.za
#eatcleantraindirty

INTRODUCTION BY DR GREG VENNING

HE WAS WALKING down the road, hand in hand with his wife to cheering crowds and worldwide press coverage. He was arguably the most famous person on the planet, not just on that day but also for the life he had led and would lead. It was the 11 February 1990 and the man was Nelson Mandela and the event his release from prison.

Growing up in South Africa at that time I learned something that was burned into my being: it is not acceptable to keep quiet about things that matter. That message has spurred me on to serve humanity.

The idea for this book germinated over many years from that desire to serve and was fertilised by Elan Lohmann. When we sat together at the Vineyard Hotel in Cape Town on the 14th February 2013 I realised I had met someone special. We have collaborated ever since and this book is the result. While these are my words you will be reading, Elan and the people of SleekGeek, his online and real life network – who want to experience vitality in their lives – have been essential in helping me get this message out. I have been working in the field of human potential for over 15 years as a sports coach, therapist, chiropractor, transformational coach and speaker and I have witnessed many transformations. In these pages I have distilled my experience and research. Thrive! promises powerful transformation of your mind-body toward vitality by giving you the why, how and what of a vitalistic lifestyle.

You have the ability to do more, love more, serve more, experience more and create more than you think you can. To get to a different result in your life you have to be prepared to do new things and the prerequisite for doing anything new in life is hope. I want you to know that you are creative, resourceful and whole. I want you to know that your mind-body has the capacity to give you all the energy you need to live a big life. I want you to know that it is not your destiny to get sick and live a life limited by your body, your state of mind or your state of health.

Yours in well-being.

Dr Greg Venning.
Cape Town
April 2016

INTRODUCTION BY ELAN LOHMANN

I FIRST SPOTTED Dr Greg on social media when my Sleekgeek community had just a few hundred members and I'm grateful to the universe that I did. We connected instantly at our first face-to-face meeting and I just knew instinctively that we could produce something valuable together; I just was not sure exactly what at the time. We soon realised that we shared a common mission to change the world and improve the health and quality of lives of as many people as we could.

I'm extremely protective of my Sleekgeek brand and community and therefore particularly selective about whom I choose to work and associate with; I don't easily partner. Dr Greg is a balanced, wise and professional individual of the highest standard. His teachings and philosophy are congruent and consistent with my personal belief system and journey.

The practices, philosophies and truths that excite and inspire me are now in your hands in the pages of this book. Thrive! is not for someone wanting to quickly lose some weight at any cost. It's not a diet guide. It's a template to become the Ultimate You.

I'm delighted that we found a way of spreading our and others' ideas through this book. It's refreshing to work with professionals like Dr Greg who base their opinions on countless hours of reading, research and experience. The ideas and teachings in Thrive! are the result of years of accumulating and making sense of information. Consequently anything Dr Greg says you can bet there is a real solid backing for it!

There is no doubt that you and the quality of your life is a result of how you eat, how you move and how you think, and that you truly have the power to make change. I wish you the happiest, healthiest life humanly possible and your achieving this would make my soul smile.

Thrive! will show you the way.

Elan Lohmann
Cape Town
April 2016

THRIVE!

Only for those who want to be healthy

DR GREG VENNING
WITH ELAN LOHMANN

First published in South Africa in 2016
by Vital Press
26 Draper Square, 14 Draper Street, Claremont, Cape Town.

ISBN: 978-0-994-6840-0-4

Packaged by Publishing Print Matters (Pty) Ltd, Cape Town
Editorial Panel: Luke Arnold and Robin Stuart-Clark
Final formatting for press: The Design Drawer

Cover Design: One Designs

Printed by Megadigital, Cape Town.

Dedication

To MP and SB – How did I get so lucky?
Love FF.

CONTENTS

THRIVE! MAP

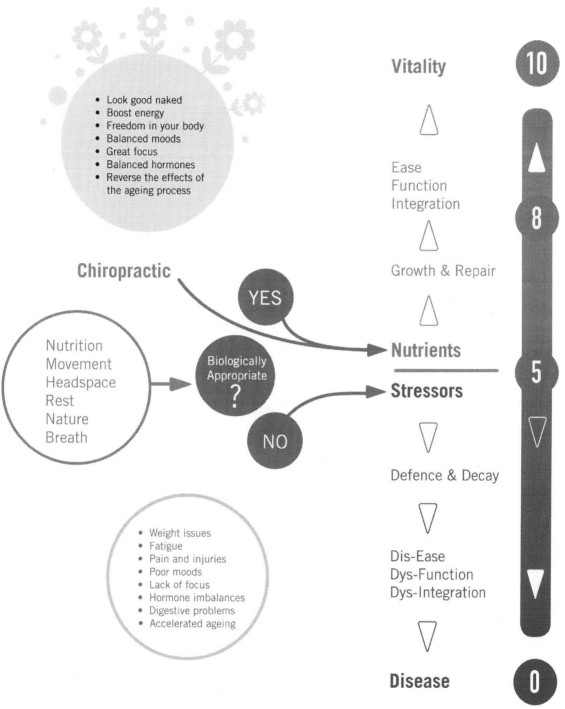

Vitality   10

- Look good naked
- Boost energy
- Freedom in your body
- Balanced moods
- Great focus
- Balanced hormones
- Reverse the effects of the ageing process

Ease
Function
Integration

8

Growth & Repair

Chiropractic

YES

Nutrition
Movement
Headspace
Rest
Nature
Breath

Biologically
Appropriate
?

Nutrients

5

Stressors

NO

Defence & Decay

- Weight issues
- Fatigue
- Pain and injuries
- Poor moods
- Lack of focus
- Hormone imbalances
- Digestive problems
- Accelerated ageing

Dis-Ease
Dys-Function
Dys-Integration

Disease   0

Dr Greg Venning   http://thrivelifestyle.solutions

1

Why vitality?

Y ou are born to be healthy and lean, to be fit, and happy. Good moods, abundant energy, great shape, balanced hormones, fantastic focus and productivity: these are coded in your genes. The only reason why we aren't where we would like to be is because of the choices we make every single day to either give our mind-body the raw materials it requires for health, or to deprive it of those raw materials.

Thrive not survive!

Most people aren't aware of this but each one of the 75 trillion cells that make up your body has only two gears. Cellular biology tells us that every cell in your body can either exist in a state of growth or a state of defence, nothing in between.

Once you realise that you are an ecosystem of these trillions of cells all organised into tissues and organs, like your liver or heart, you too can either be in growth or defence, survival mode or thrive mode. You're either moving forward or you're moving backwards.

Being in survival mode means that the best that you generally feel is just 'ok'. You may not be sick but you're certainly not at your best: your mind and body may be a little stiffer than they should be; you may be carrying a little extra weight around your middle; your moods and energy are up and down; and because there's nothing apparently wrong, you're 'healthy'. Consequently, in this state you may not be sick but you certainly aren't performing at your best. At worst, being in survival mode essentially means that you have a condition or disease that is seriously compromising your health and your ability to lead a full, active, happy life.

Moving yourself from a state of survival to one of thriving opens up a new world of possibilities where innate but dormant forces, faculties and abilities are activated.

In Thrive! mode you'll begin to access your potential to live a bigger life, where being lean is normal, where having energy is par for the course. In Thrive! mode you enjoy freedom and confidence in your body, you find it easy to manage your weight and you enjoy your good moods and have balanced hormones. Focus and productivity are by-products of Thrive! When you Thrive! you move beyond just being healthy into a higher gear: Vitality.

WHAT'S YOUR POTENTIAL? How much of it are you sacrificing everyday for the sake of the status quo? For the sake of 'comfort'? Living a life of average proportions

CASE HISTORY 1:
A story of survive to Thrive!

A FEW YEARS ago Linda (not her real name), came to my practice. She was experiencing severe back pain after picking up her son just a few days before. Linda also told me that she had headaches all day, every day. "I just thought that was normal," she told me. When I said that having a headache all day, every day was certainly not normal she could hardly believe me. For all her adult life, Linda had been living with this pain which became part of her existence, part of her 'normal.'

After a period of care with us Linda's headaches eased and became less frequent. "I can think clearer, I have more energy, I can be a better mom," she said with tears in her eyes. "I can't believe that I thought that my headaches were normal!"

With a few lifestyle modifications and some time to let her mind-body heal, Linda improved even more: she was down a few dress sizes and more energetic. She was living a bigger life, one she thought she could never have. "Doc, I'm 40 and this is the best I've felt since I was 20!"

Linda's story is not uncommon. Lots of us learn to live sub-par lives because we see other people doing it. We learn to think that average is normal and that we shouldn't expect too much from our well-being. We learn mediocrity, in fact, we are hypnotised by it and consequently silently sacrifice our life's potential.

is not comfortable, it's painful but, invariably, it's a pain you have learned to live with because you thought there was no alternative.

The essence of Thrive! is to help you to live a life bursting with energy. The idea is to help you to look good naked, move with freedom, have balanced moods, boost energy, be connected with your purpose in life, be able to raise healthier kids, be fit for life, be able to lose that middle age spread and do it all while having a blast!

Making a fresh start

et me share some truths with you. These truths are all around you but you probably aren't aware of them; I know I wasn't.

These truths have the potential to reactivate something within you, something you've been looking for – perhaps even subconsciously. You may be looking for more energy, better focus, better control of your weight or address some kind of ache, pain or medical condition. You may be looking to take your personal performance to the next level and to achieve something great. But you feel you just can't.

I know this because I went through the same thing. I had a yearning to be more, do more, feel more alive and to experience more life. The way I experienced life was pretty typical. I was unhappy on a deep level but outwardly I seemed fine. I had the surface challenges many of us have: I was overweight despite trying to eat well and exercise; I had mood and energy issues; I had bouts of depression and I didn't do well in relationships; I was having mediocre professional success even though my peers held me in high esteem. Outwardly it seemed like things were good but inwardly I was living a small and unfulfilled life.

Living a bigger life will mean different things to each of us but innately we are all looking for the things that will make us happiest. You and I are always acting in ways that we think will bring us happiness, doing things that we think will give us the next high, the next bit of peace or the next moment of excitement. Even when we do stupid things that sabotage our progress, we do it out of some deep, unconscious sense that it will help us. You are creative, resourceful and whole and you are doing the best you can with the hand you've been dealt.

As I discovered and tested these truths, I began to change; not just change but really transform. My body transformed – the fat came off and I built muscle, my skin cleared up, my sinus problems disappeared and I felt more freedom in my body. I found that I really loved movement, that I craved it and felt my best when I was expressing myself through movement. I felt more alive and connected with my body than I ever had.

My mind transformed and my energy levels improved. The constant internal chatter of my ego started to diminish, the mood swings began to balance and my concentration and focus just skyrocketed. I felt more present, more aware and more creative than I had ever felt.

Since my vocation is to help others I began to share these insights and truths with my friends and family. People asked me what I had done to look so much better so I started coaching them, too. I was in practice at the time and so I shared my insights with my practice members. As each of the people around me began to implement the very same principles I used, they also began to change. Some changed faster than others and some needed more help than others. Sometimes we had to find different solutions for people and I realised that it wasn't a 'one size fits all' application the principles however, were universal.

Soon I was coaching individuals and groups, internationally on Skype and locally in person. Next was a series of seminars where people had powerful transformative experiences. For each person I worked with there is a unique set of challenges and as long as we were honest with each other and stuck to the principles, we achieved change.

I will be your imperfect guide. I don't pretend to be perfect, because I have my challenges, just like you. I fall down and I get lost. I act small and I get hurt. From my own personal experience and those whom I have coached, I know I can help you to get the more out of our experience of life. What you will learn here is how to make the seemingly impossible, possible – and Thrive!

Why should you read this book?

THRIVE! is based on the premise that you are inherently well, healthy and whole. You have an innate ability to self-develop, self-regulate, heal and express your health at the highest levels. Contrary to what you might have been taught or think, you are not broken.

THRIVE! will help you to make a transformational shift for a lifetime while making some good short term progress too.

THRIVE! will take you beyond yet another diet, exercise plan or positive thinking method and help you to incorporate the three essential requirements for well-being – Nutrition, Movement and Headspace – and begin to create a lifestyle for a lifetime.

Whether you are already healthy and looking to access higher levels of personal performance or you're not feeling your best and want to improve, or even if you have health challenges and you want your life back, Thrive! can help you make this happen.

THRIVE! is not another new fad; it draws on the best, most effective ways to move toward a lifestyle of vitality based on human biology. These principles are scientifically sound and have been used effectively by many people across the globe.

THRIVE! relies on the best that the science of wellness has to offer and answers two of the most fundamental questions you could ever ask yourself:

What is my potential?
How do I achieve lifelong vitality?

Using the universal principles of human behaviour Thrive! explores how you got to where you are now and how you can do things differently to get to where you would prefer to be. Many of us don't actually know where we want to be and Thrive! will help you to address this critical issue, too.

Unlike the things you've tried in the past, Thrive! will help you make the required emotional and mental shift to achieve real lifestyle change.

You're going to find that your beliefs and assumptions about well-being and what is 'healthy' will be challenged. I won't tell you to 'eat less', 'exercise more' or 'think positively'.

Instead of telling you how you can temporarily cover symptoms and just lose weight or just increase energy or just create focus or just manage stress, Thrive! asks how you can activate your innate potential for vitality and reap all the weight management, energy, fitness and focus rewards in the process.

When you focus on small things like just losing weight or beating stress you can often miss the bigger picture. While weight and energy are the things that are bothering you there is something larger at stake. If all you ever focus on is the puddle on the floor you'll never address the leak in the roof. Thrive! is not a 'puddle on the floor' kind of book. Thrive! questions the 'leak in the roof' and offers a way to repair it so it doesn't leak again.

6

What Thrive! offers is a checklist for creating health, and sustaining vitality.

Instead of only looking at diet or exercise or mental and emotional stress, we will look at the whole picture. Dealing with just one or two of these issues can be helpful in the short term, but without a complete picture you'll never live up to your full potential and you will risk developing a serious disease.

You'll find real examples of how many people have practised Thrive! principles and the difference Thrive! has made in their lives.

The solutions Thrive! provides will challenge many of your currently held beliefs. Right now your state of health is a result of your beliefs. Your beliefs form your mental blueprint of the world, what is and isn't possible and what you are and aren't willing to do. These beliefs are mostly unconscious but guide every decision you make every day and your daily decisions determine your destiny.

How is Thrive! different from other books?

You're going to find that your beliefs and assumptions about well-being and what is 'healthy' will be challenged. You won't hear us tell you to 'eat less' 'exercise more' or 'think positively' in this book. What you will find are scientifically sound strategies and tactics that have been proven to work in the real world for real people, just like you.

This books asks a different question to many others. Instead of asking how we can temporarily cover symptoms and just lose weight or just increase energy or just create focus or just manage stress, this book asks how we can activate our innate potential for vitality and reap all the weight management, energy, fitness and focus rewards in the process.

That means that you won't find any sections here on how to address specific symptoms. We aren't claiming to treat or cure any disease or condition. What you'll get in the following pages is a checklist for creating health and as you follow that checklist you'll be surprised at the results you can achieve.

That means that we have been able to put together a comprehensive, integrated approach to well-being instead of a fragmented one. That means that this might be the first time you've ever had the chance to put the pieces of the puzzle together and realise your true potential.

When we look at what lifestyle choices create health, we've questioned the status quo and conventional wisdom. We've gone back to the drawing board and looked at our movement, nutrition and headspace through the wide angle lens of biology and evolution. We've then applied and lived these lessons for ourselves and helped others to do the same. There is nothing in this book that we have not done for ourselves.

We'll also give you real life examples of how lots of people have put our principles into practice and how much of a difference it has made in their lives. These principles work and they can work for you.

In this book we're putting the pieces of the wellness lifestyle puzzle together for you, probably for the first time. By looking at ourselves in a very different way from the way we usually do we've been able to define what our mind-body biologically requires for well-being.

You don't have to take our word for it. Do some research and ask some questions for yourself. Just be careful which questions you ask ...

What difference will Thrive! make in my life?

Your state of health right now has little to do with bad luck, bad germs or bad genes. It has everything to do with the choices you make every day. You are not a victim of your circumstances, you are the pilot, you are the navigator and you are in charge. The choices you've made up until now haven't been for lack of will power or good intentions.

You have the potential for greatness – to live a full life and to experience amazing things, to create value for yourself and for others, to help and care for those around you: we all do. You have the potential to have loads of energy, to feel good about how you look, to have a mind-body that performs well, not just for now, but for life. It might seem like an unrealistic dream for you. You might think that these are the things that only lucky people can experience and achieve. I used to think the same way.

The sense of balance, strength, freedom and power that comes from a mind-body existing in a state of well-being is our birthright. Vitality is a state of personal and physiological growth and repair, where we are more resistant to stress and disease and are capable of handling our daily stressors with a sense of ease. We can learn to dance in the chaos of life and Thrive!

This state of being – our vitality – is our default setting. To re-activate it we have to look to the source and not just change but TRANSFORM.

Why are questions so important?

The quality of your life is determined by the quality of your questions.
JOHN DEMARTINI

Our view of the world is constructed by the questions we ask. Questions reveal the nature of the universe to us. Shine a torch on an object in a dark room from one angle and it can look like a monster. Shining the torch from a different angle, however, can reveal that the monster is just a coat hanging on a door. The answers revealed depend on the questions asked.

If you are experiencing pain and wonder, "How do I make myself feel better as quickly as possible?", your answer is a painkiller. That painkiller only masks the problem for a while until the problem resurfaces. The problem was not caused by a lack of a painkiller in the first place. If you ask, "How can I heal myself?", you will find answers that address the underlying causes: for example, addressing structural misalignments, undergoing rehabilitation, making sure your body has all the nutrients it needs to heal and, of course, believing it will happen. ●

The groundwork of all happiness is health.
JAMES LEIGH HUNT

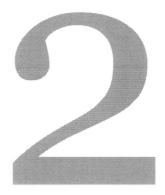

Health is sick and wellness has sold out

What is our current definition of health?

> *It is clear, then, that in the science of nature as elsewhere,*
> *we should try first to determine questions about the first principles.*
> ARISTOTLE

Health as it's defined by the World Health Organisation is **"a state of complete physical, mental, and social well-being and not merely the absence of disease or infirmity."** Unfortunately this is not the meaning of the word 'health' as we use it today. Today 'health' simply means that we're not sick. Health has come to mean only 'the absence of disease or infirmity'.

This change in thinking is hurting us and I'll show you how: rate your health on a scale of 0-10, where 10 is your optimum potential. Obviously most people aren't going to fit each of these score descriptions exactly, so rate yourself according to the one that best matches your level of health. Be brutally honest with yourself.

8-10 – HAVING A ZEST FOR LIFE, being vibrant and energetic, being connected to your purpose in life, being in peak physical health, having great moods and boundless energy every day, feeling good about how you look, enjoying restful sleep and waking up without an alarm clock.

7 – YOUR ENERGY LEVELS ARE MORE UP THAN DOWN; your stress levels will get the best of you from time to time. Sleep is not a problem but you do wake up tired more often than you'd like. Physically you might feel strong some of the time but you're nowhere near your best and you may be carrying extra weight that is tough to budge. Mentally you feel alright but there is the occasional brain fog and memory lapse, and your sense of purpose is unclear sometimes.

5 – A NEUTRAL POINT at which there is nothing really wrong but nothing right, either. Around 5 your energy will be lower than you'd like; you may have rings under your eyes regularly and have more than occasional problems getting restful sleep. You might have a spare tire around your waist or thighs and occasional minor aches, pains or other symptoms like heartburn, period pains, digestive issues, headaches, sinus trouble – possibly with acute episodes. Mentally and emotionally you're up and down with what society might consider 'normal' brain fog and memory issues and there is no clear sense of purpose in your life.

3 – YOU ARE NOTICEABLY FATIGUED and usually have some difficulty getting restful sleep – the rings under your eyes tell a story. Stress levels are moderate to high and feelings of irritability, anxiety or depression are noticeable. Physically you have more days with aches, pains or other symptoms with frequent acute episodes. Your moods would be more down than up and you'd have a distinct lack of connectedness or purpose in your life.

0 – CRISIS. Constant fatigue and exhaustion with poor sleep and stress levels would be pushing you to within inches of your breaking point. You'll have some form of chronic pain or illness with frequent acute episodes. Mentally and emotionally you would experience severe depression or anxiety. This is the worst you could imagine yourself without being dead!

I've done this exercise with thousands of people from all over the world and the most common responses are between levels 5 and 7. When I ask if they are 'healthy' the answer is 'yes'. They believe they are healthy simply because there is nothing specifically wrong. They have the second part of the WHO definition of health, 'the absence of disease or infirmity', but they are not in a 'a state of complete physical, mental, and social well-being'. This state only occurs between levels 8 and 10. There is a lot more to being healthy than not being sick and living in the 5-7 range leads to a life of average proportions. Our understanding of the word 'health' has lost half of its meaning and it is a significant loss.

Limiting beliefs

When did it become normal for us to live at 5-7/10 and call ourselves healthy? When did it become normal for us to sacrifice at least 30% of our potential for a vibrant and energetic life? When did we start teaching our children that missing out on the top 50% of their potential for health was normal or even acceptable? When did we begin to think that not being sick means you are healthy? Surely there is more to life than not being sick?

Consequently, we now think it's normal to get chronically ill as we get older. Diseases that hardly existed 100 years ago are now the industrialised world's biggest killers: obesity, diabetes, cancer, heart disease, chronic pain, depression and anxiety – to name just a few – are so prevalent now that they seem normal but they were all relatively unknown 100 years ago. 80% of all lost productivity in the industrialised world's workforce is because of at least one chronic, degenerative, incurable disease.

In northern Thailand a few years ago my wife and I saw an elephant with a mahout (handler). It was a big elephant bull tethered by a leash to a stake in the ground. He was swaying from side to side and turning his head which I knew from my holidays spent camping in the bush, was a sign of distress. What was curious to us was that the stake in the ground was no bigger than a broomstick. There was no way that this fragile stick in the ground would hold this elephant if he really wanted to be somewhere else.

We asked the mahout about this and why the big bull, clearly agitated, stayed where he was. The mahout told us how he and the elephant had been together for over 30 years and how, when the bull had been a young calf, it had been tied to a similar stake. No matter how much the young calf pulled, the stake held fast and he couldn't get free.

Now that the elephant had grown into a large bull – an amazingly powerful creature – he still saw this stake as something that held him, no matter how much he might have wanted to get away.

If we've been brought up to think that 7/10 is fine and anything more is too hard to accomplish or downright impossible, then that belief is going to hold us there like a stake, tethering us to the ground. Even more saddening is that we're going to pass this belief on to our children, because they learn from what we do and not from what we say.

The journey

We can view our well-being as a journey that each of us is on. When we begin our journey at birth, we have a very high level of health expression and potential – barring any problems with birth or pregnancy, babies are generally very healthy. There are two factors that, as we grow and develop, are going to affect us and determine what level of health we will express.

1. STRESSORS: these are the things that create imbalance in your mind-body, things that bring your level of health down, that break you down over time. Stressors are evident in three main forms:
   - MENTAL/EMOTIONAL – work, family, finances, relationships, keeping a household running, studying or even loss of a loved one.

- CHEMICAL – things we put into or onto our body from food and drink to drugs (prescribed and pushed) and smoking. It also includes the chemicals in our food, cosmetics, air and water.
- PHYSICAL – injuries and accidents, the exercise we do or the exercise we aren't doing, sitting for long hours each day.

2. RESISTANCE: While these stressors are breaking you down you have an ability to heal and regulate yourself, which we call our Innate Resistance. It allows you to survive these stressors, to fight infections, to resist disease and to grow and regenerate. Some time ago I cut my right hand while playing in a tree. The cut healed and there is no scar because my body has healed: this is our Innate Resistance.

If I decide I want to eat just one cheeseburger I probably won't die of a heart attack right there and then. That's because my mind-body can resist the stress that one cheeseburger can cause.

If your accumulated stressors are matched by your level of resistance then you will maintain a high level of health expression. But if you accumulate more stressors than your mind-body can resist, then you're in the process of being broken down. Now this is usually a slow process and because we generally live our lives day to day, we hardly notice the breakdown. In fact we think it's normal because we see others experiencing the same thing.

If someone was behind you slowly dimming the lights in your room, your eyes would compensate for the fading light. If this was done slowly enough it might be so subtle that you wouldn't notice it. Now your mind-body has to compensate for the breakdown caused by chronic stressors over time just like your eyes adjust with poor light. As your mind-body compensates or adapts to the lower levels of light you suffer a loss of function that you usually can't feel. In the poor light you might realise you can't see as far or are unable to read the small text. In this process of mind-body breakdown you might also notice you have lower levels of energy, poor mobility, memory issues or weight gain.

While you accumulate stressors your mind-body adapts until it gets to a point where compensation no longer works. At this point you cross a line and begin to develop symptoms like pain or heartburn or restricted movement or decreased energy or anxiety or weight gain. What we usually do then is seek the help of a health care professional of some sort, be it a medical doctor, a Chiropractor, a physiotherapist, a homeopath or another health professional, and look for a 'magic bullet' solution.

For example you have a headache and go to see your doctor. What would your doctor likely give you to relieve a headache? Probably a painkiller of some sort. You take the pill and expect the headache to go away. But was the headache caused by the lack of a painkiller in your body? It's a question that sounds quite odd and most of the people I've asked look slightly bemused and say, "Of course not!" Yet we continue to do what we've always done, as if the pill will magically remove the problem – until the next time.

The problem will recur, maybe as a headache or some other kind of symptom. We'll most likely do the same thing and find a quick fix to cover the problem. And if we've done it twice we're likely to do it over and over again to numb the pain. The problem with doing this repeatedly is that each time you drop below the line you do more irreparable damage to the tissues of your body. As long as we feel little or no discomfort in the process then we think that it's fine.

We usually do this until we've done so much damage that we can't get relief anymore. Drugs and surgery can't help us and we're left to make what we can with the end of our lives.

This is the medical model we follow nowadays called 'health care'. We know that there is more to being healthy than not being sick so I suggest that we call this 'sickcare'. The 'sickcare' system is perfect for dealing with emergencies but if you entrust your well-being to such a system you will live a life of average proportions.

Under the hood

The driving beliefs that underlie the 'sickcare' model of health are:

Not sick = healthy

- **BELIEF** – a lack of symptoms is the same as being healthy and treating a symptom makes you healthier.
- **HOW YOU ACT** – If you have high cholesterol all you need is a pill to drive down the high cholesterol, without thinking about what causes it to go up. Once the cholesterol number is down, you think you're fine.

- **HOW YOU THINK** – You believe that eliminating the symptom is the same as addressing the cause. You think that the high cholesterol number on the blood test was the real problem and once it's down you believe you're healthy.

EXAMPLE – putting a plaster on the 'low oil' warning light on the dashboard of your car and thinking that you've solved the problem

You are a machine

- **BELIEF** – you are reducible to the sum of your parts that can be separated, altered, removed or replaced.
- **HOW YOU ACT** – You take a drug to alter the way your liver works and so produce less cholesterol and don't consider the underlying cause or how the pill affects the rest of your body.
- **HOW YOU THINK** – you ignore the fact that there are many things that affect cholesterol levels and that it's not just the liver. You think that by taking the pill you are fixing your broken liver and are unaware that the drug stops your liver from creating important chemicals, also affects your other organs and can cause more harm than good.

EXAMPLE – after the Second World War we began spraying the toxic chemical DDT over crops to kill pests. Only decades later we realised the detrimental effect it had on the entire ecosystem downstream, affecting many plants and animals and almost driving species like the Bald Eagle into extinction.

You are broken

- **BELIEF** – your body is inherently flawed and needs outside intervention to fix it.
- **HOW YOU ACT** – when you become aware of a problem you use drugs or surgery to chemically or physically alter the 'broken' part.
- **HOW YOU THINK** – you think your body is inherently flawed and liable to breaking down and only drugs or surgeries can fix them.

EXAMPLE – covering the vent of your air-conditioner because it's blowing too cold on your neck instead of realising that the thermostat is sensing the rise in temperature because the cold air is escaping through the open window: you think that something is broken (air-conditioner) and you only address the effect (vent) and not the cause (the window).

You are separate from nature

- **BELIEF** – you are not an animal and not subject to natural laws.
- **HOW YOU ACT** – when someone gets cancer, hardly any attention is paid to the person's lifestyle or their environment. I've heard 'world renowned experts' telling cancer patients that diet and exercise patterns won't affect their disease at all.
- **HOW YOU THINK** – you can ruin your health through poor lifestyle and then hope a drug, lotion, potion or surgery will be invented to fix it.

EXAMPLE – when we sprayed DDT on our crops and didn't realise it would affect us. People who consumed crops sprayed with DDT suffered miscarriages, pre-term birth, early weaning and fertility issues in men and women and there are further links to cancer.

What are the consequences?

The consequences of 'sickcare' could not be more severe. As a society and as individuals we are sacrificing our potential at the altar of mediocrity just so that we can feel some temporary comfort. This loss of our human potential happens so slowly and gradually that we hardly notice it. We make compromise after compromise and slowly erode our personal performance and then wonder why we feel so wrung out, so tired, so sick and why our children get so sick.

Two primary consequences are:
1. **Chronic disease** like cancer, heart disease, diabetes, obesity, chronic pain, depression, anxiety, learning disorders, Alzheimers.
2. **The loss of your potential** to live a bigger life in 'pre-disease' states where you might not feel any symptoms and your mind-body is underperforming.

The black plague killed 30% of the population of Europe. In industrialised societies like the US and Europe, 80% of people will have a chronic, degenerative, 'incurable' disease during their lives! Of this 80%, many will have two or more of these diseases. This statistic does not apply to the elderly, but rather to people 35-65 years old!

Today, chronic diseases are seen in children at an alarming rate. Learning problems, autism, allergies, diabetes, obesity, early puberty, depression and anxiety are all on the rise in children and young people. Diseases we once thought were relegated to the old age home are now evident in schools and kindergartens.

Why should you care?

When you are faced with global statistics of diseases they generally don't mean much because the voice in your head says, "I'm ok. That won't happen to me." A loss of health generally happens gradually, so what signs might you see early on that would warn you that you are on a path of average, limited proportions?

Consider this: you are awakened by your alarm clock or children most mornings, not particularly refreshed. Either the quality of your sleep, or the number of hours you were able to sleep, doesn't seem to recharge you the way it used to. If you're lucky you're out of bed without any aches or stiffness though, more often than not, you have to gingerly peel yourself off the mattress and move slowly because of a painful back, neck, hip, shoulder, knee etc.

You rush through your morning routine that probably includes a stimulant like caffeine to get you up and functional. Maybe you have breakfast, maybe not, and then everyone's out of the house. But, if you're like most people, before you leave home there is a 1 in 4 chance that your children are on a prescription medication and a 4 in 5 chance that you will require a prescription pill or dose during the day. This statistic rises even more if you add in over the counter drugs.

During your average day, without possibly realising, you will experience some early sign of the onset of a chronic disease. Maybe it's heartburn, energy dips and mood swings, aches and pains, skin conditions like eczema or acne, generally low mood or brain fog.

A long, hard look in a mirror would reveal one or more signs of breakdown, like dark rings under the eyes, poor posture, spare tyres that haven't budged despite numerous diets, cellulite, varicose veins, skin blemishes or sagging muscles.

A recent diet challenge might have been moderately successful but not enough to motivate you to stick to it beyond a couple of months. You might have also noticed that you aren't recovering from exercise as quickly as you used to and with recurrent injuries it's more difficult to fit exercise into your 'busy' schedule.

Menstrual pain is a common problem for many women and cycles may even be irregular. Conditions like endometriosis, PCOS and infertility are frighteningly common amongst many women today.

You and your partner will have probably experienced some sexual dysfunction or loss of libido more regularly than you'd care to admit. Male infertility is also alarmingly prevalent today.

Gas, bloating, constipation and diarrhoea become so regular that you think it's normal without realising that these conditions could be early signs of chronic disease. Food intolerance – to wheat, dairy etc. – and allergies may also start to play a role.

Getting through most days is a chore with significant energy dips and accompanying mood swings that are managed by snacking or bingeing or drinking more stimulants like tea (green tea as well), coffee and energy drinks. Daily life has become so pressurised that alcohol or smoking as a way of 'winding down' has become a nightly habit.

Do any of these things sound familiar to you? Even with all these indicators of harmful living most people don't realise what they're doing to themselves. We think these are minor, temporary issues and that they can be overcome when we're ready. The trouble is we don't overcome them because the process of harm is already in motion.

We are not very good at understanding and applying this type of information and extending it into the future. Something about how we think about the future and the way we process this information doesn't seem to be any good in helping us plan for the future. No matter how many times we hear financial experts telling us to begin saving for retirement, we don't. No matter how much we are told we're damaging our planet we don't seem to change the way we treat our environment.

Now consider the cost of all of these seemingly mild complaints in your life in relation to what they actually mean to you today.

What does your fatigue cost you every day?

When you are groggy, sore or distracted, what are you missing out on at home? The giggling of your kids, that great sunset, your spouse's request that somehow gets forgotten and leads to yet another argument? Do your gut issues, joint pains, fatigue, energy slumps, low moods and brain fog make you no fun to be around?

These are all very real things for you, even though you don't realise it. At work you miss deadlines, forget emails and generally don't work at the level that you'd like to or you're expected to. Somehow you always feel like you're one step behind everyone else and struggling to catch up. Consequently you spend more time on work-related things and you miss out on your family and social life.

Are you deeply unhappy about the state of your body and what you see in the mirror, despite the brave face you put on? Do you shy away from many potentially exciting and fulfilling opportunities for fear of these blemishes being noticed, or for fear of not being able to cope physically with the demands?

If any of these issues sound familiar to you there is a lot you can do about it, starting now! We find that these things are largely preventable and reversible when we begin to ask new questions.

The cost of 'health'

No one wants to be the healthiest corpse in the grave and often the road to 'health' is thought to be one of starvation and deprivation. The fastest way for a restaurant to stop selling an item on their menu is to label it as the 'Healthy Option.' One of the missing links in most health care messages is, "What's in it for me?"

None of the financial crises we've experienced and none of the wars we've fought come close to how much our health crisis is hurting us. This is not just my opinion, but the opinion of a growing number of health authorities around the globe.

The emerging problem is so big that in 2011 the UN held a special session worthy of a full general assembly of most of the world's leaders to discuss the issue. The last time they thought something was this important was when they convened to discuss the HIV/AIDS issue. In this meeting many leaders said that the effects of chronic, non-communicable diseases far exceeds that caused by HIV/AIDS.

The Collective Cost

The financial cost of the 'sickcare' system is staggering. Our current paradigm of thought says, "If I don't have symptoms then I'm not sick", which is one of the main reasons why we're in the midst of this crisis right now. This way of thinking is similar to that which would make you wait until you had a toothache before you started brushing your teeth. This is the type of thinking that has allowed the chronic health crisis to develop in the first place. Dr Chan, the Director-General of the WHO, called this crisis a 'slow motion disaster' and an 'ominous wave for which the prognosis is grim'. The fact remains, however, that the disaster is speeding up.

The statistics in the United Nations report are compelling. 63% of global deaths (of the 57 million in 2010) were due to chronic, preventable diseases. By 2030 it will be 52 million deaths every year. Treatment of diabetes alone accounts for 15% of national budgets in some countries and health care spending in the US will reach $4.3 trillion by 2017.

Let's give that number the respect that it deserves: $4 300 000 000 000.00. This is what treating these diseases in one country for one year would cost. It's such a big number, I can't even fit it in my calculator, let alone comprehend it, so let's put it in perspective: it's $12 billion a day and $8 million a minute!

What's not being factored in here is the amount of lost productivity that we would experience. When people are sick, they are off work more frequently and, even if they are at work, they aren't as productive as they could be. Chronic disease causes an 80% decrease in productivity in people of working age. This lack of productivity was estimated to result in a loss of $47 trillion from the global economy from 2011-2013. It is enough money to eliminate poverty for the poorest 2,5 billion people in the world right now.

What is truly frightening is that these reports are probably underestimates because they were only talking about 'The Big Four' chronic diseases – cancer, cardiovascular disease, diabetes and chronic respiratory disease. Those figures don't mention mental health, which alongside cardiovascular disease is the leading type of chronic disease, and costs £105 billion in the UK alone. Also not mentioned are musculoskeletal conditions ranging from back pain (the most common cause of time off work costing billions a year) to arthritis, auto-immune conditions from multiple sclerosis and celiac disease to eczema and lupus.

The monetary cost is so big that even though I try to put it into context, I still can't fathom the true extent of the cost. The sense that I get from all these dizzying numbers is that this 'ominous wave' is already affecting global prosperity. It is shaping our financial markets and stunting growth in ways that are affecting decisions made at the highest level far more that other market forces, such as the price of gold or oil or the value of the US dollar.

The Individual Cost

The monetary cost pales in comparison to the real cost, however. How I interpret all of this data is on a much more personal and simplistic level. The 'slow motion disaster' of chronic disease that we are in right now is shaping our lives and those of our children and our grandchildren. I'm confident it has shaped a fair amount of your life already. Have you known someone who has had a heart attack? Someone who has battled cancer? Has a stroke affected you or someone you know? How about obesity, depression, diabetes, arthritis, chronic anxiety or chronic fatigue? The question I should be asking is whether anyone hasn't been affected by any of these conditions.

When these conditions affect the lives of adults, we experience a significant decrease in quality of life. Over the years patients have told me that they have to budget their energy every day and consequently miss out on a lot of living. Not only do they feel like spectators in the game of life but they feel disempowered financially; they can't work because of their health or they are paying a large portion of their income to 'sickcare' costs. Chronic conditions may also affect the future earning potential of families by taking one parent early or handicapping them.

This does not just apply to elderly people. 80% of time taken off work with chronic diseases is by people between 35 and 60 years of age. Apart from suicide, heart disease and cancer are the two most common causes of death for people 15-34 years old in the US. These diseases start in childhood; they are not diseases of old age.

Not only are more people getting sicker in old age and tapping into our health resources, but there are more and more people of working age who are ill and tapping into those resources while not contributing to them as much as they should. In addition to this, younger people entering into the work force are sicker than ever, meaning that they also drain our resources and will contribute less than the generations before them. This is a sick system: it consumes more than it produces but it's what we call our 'health care system'.

The loss of quality of life for every person affects me deeply, none more so than when it affects children. Our way of living is damaging our children's biology in disturbing ways. Girls and boys are beginning puberty at earlier and earlier ages and it is now common to find signs of spinal decay and degeneration by the age of 15. How much of life are they going to miss out on because these conditions will dull their vitality, bring down their energy and shorten their lives?

My primary concern, however, is the loss of human potential that comes with our global state of ill-being.

The innate potential brought to the world with the birth of a child is amazing. Imagining what a child or adult's potential to create and experience in their life leaves me in a state of awe. How much love could you experience? Could you make people stop in their tracks with your art? How much joy could you create? Could you help people to discover far flung places? Could you be a caring doctor to those who need you? Could you live a fulfilling life and enjoy your retirement years playing golf and enjoying the fruits of your labour? Could that child have so much love for a sport that they earn a living from it? Could that little girl eventually become a nurturing mother? Could that 20 year old open a new company that creates value for millions of people? It's the realisation of that potential that embodies my definition of vitality and it's the loss of that potential that drives me.

You are born with the potential to live an extraordinary life, to be fulfilled and to contribute to the evolution of mankind. More than ever, that pool of potential that exists amongst us, that could create so much, is threatening to go untapped. It's being wasted, squandered and lost. Our ability to live great lives, to create amazing things, to shape an amazing future is under serious threat and it has serious and very personal consequences.

What about the children?
A friend of mine is a primary school teacher and she estimates that about 1 in 2 of the children between the ages of 10-12 are on a prescription medication for learning and behaviour of some sort. Her estimates match that of a study from US where over 50% of children surveyed had used at least one medication in the preceeding 7 days. How can this be normal? Are we really this broken?

Perverse incentive

The 'sick care' system that exists right now is built on a premise that isn't working. The premise is built on 4 myths that need addressing and transformation.

    MYTH 1 – Not sick = healthy

    MYTH 2 – You are a machine

    MYTH 3 – You are broken

    MYTH 4 – You are separate from nature

'Sick care' has created a huge industry that is very useful in emergency and trauma care but not effective in addressing chronic issues. Drugs and surgery can be lifesavers in certain situations but can also be devastating in others. When we look at that system and what it costs us in human lives, things are put into perspective.

- The medical system is the 3rd leading cause of death in the UK
- The medical system is the number one cause of death and injury in the US
- 1,5 million people a year are injured by medication in the US
- The benefits of US health care may not outweigh the harm it imparts
- The 'yearly medical' with your doctor doesn't make a difference.

The disease centered 'sickcare' system is called 'allopathic' medicine and is a real lifesaver in acute and traumatic situations. Get in a car crash, have a stroke or break a leg and you are probably fortunate enough to have access to some truly wonderful doctors and nurses using amazing technology that can save limbs and lives.

The clinical practice of allopathic medicine has validity and I'm not questioning the intentions of the many amazing men and women who help countless people, sometimes in very challenging circumstances. It's the beliefs system that it's built on, the politics and the economics that drive it that I am questioning.

The allopathic mindset works in some situations, just as the fire department is good at putting out fires. The fire department has axes and hoses with water and these are great tools for bashing down doors and killing flames, but what if you wanted to prevent fires? What if houses that were neglected start to catch fire? Would it make sense to send some firemen with their axes and hoses to get to work on a house that, because of its state of neglect, is a fire risk but is not yet on fire? Is bashing down doors and spraying water going to improve the state of the derelict house?

Maybe it would make more sense to send in some contractors to work on the plumbing, electrics and structure of the place. Maybe what's needed is some tender loving care and maintenance instead of shock and awe. When it comes to chronic, degenerative diseases the allopathic mindset, like the fire department, has certain tools that might not be the right ones for the job at hand. Just like the hammers and nails of the contractors are likely to help the neglected house and axes and hoses are likely to hurt it, so drugs and surgery are probably not the right tools for dealing with chronic, degenerative conditions.

False Positives

If what we're saying sounds radical then consider these facts:

- Common procedures for heart disease, called angioplasties and stents, do not prolong life in stable individuals
- Heart bypass surgery prolongs life in less than 2-3% of patients who receive it
- Aggressive lowering of blood sugar with drugs in diabetics actually causes deaths
- "We are arguably worse off than we were in 1812", says diabetes specialist Dr. Polonsky in the New England Journal of Medicine
- The contribution of chemotherapy to survival in cancer patients is under 3%
- One third of health care expenditure in the US results in zero benefit.

No amount of drugs and surgery are going to correct the problems that a poor lifestyle can create. You can't out-medicate poor nutrition, poor movement and poor headspace.

The tools that are likely to help us in chronic, degenerative conditions are the equivalent of hammers and nails: lifestyle is equal to how we eat and drink, how we move and how we think and feel.

> *The doctor of the future will give no medicine, but will interest her or his patients in the care of the human frame, in a proper diet, and in the cause and prevention of disease.*
> THOMAS EDISON

If Edison was right then our state of health care doesn't seem to have progressed much since he died in 1931. The tools are much the same although they might be fancier, shinier and more expensive, but they remain the same tools underneath. What has changed is that care of the 'human frame' has become a profession all of it's own: Chiropractic and it fits within a vitalistic lifestyle beautifully.

There is much vested interest by the people who make the axes and hoses in the current 'sickcare' system. In a private conversation with an oncologist a few years ago, he quipped that cancer was too profitable a disease to ever cure. I hope he's wrong. I'm betting that with the emergence of the wellness paradigm we will see a whole new industry develop around creating health and not treating disease.

What is our common definition of wellness?

G iven all the trouble we're in, the wellness movement should be an answer to our troubles. It's about being proactive, about getting healthy, losing weight, getting in shape and managing stress, right?

Conventional wellness can be summed up in 5 words: **eat less and exercise more**. This mantra is nothing new, Hippocrates, father of medicine, who died in 370 BC said, "It is very injurious to health to take in more food than the constitution will bear, when, at the same time one uses no exercise to carry off this excess."

The wellness industry has boomed with diets, exercise routines, meditation retreats and the like. Everywhere you look, you will see the word 'wellness' on exercise equipment, food replacement shakes, yoga studios and book covers. In his 2007 bestselling book, *The Wellness Revolution*, Paul Zane Pilzner called it the next trillion dollar industry. Companies now have 'wellness days', medical aids encourage us to go to gym and eat healthily and give us loyalty awards, but what good has this done?

Of anyone who starts a diet, less than 5% of people are still on it 2 years later. Of anyone who starts going to a gym only 15% of people are still going at the end of the year, more than a couple of times a week. Since the advent of low-fat diets we're eating less and less of the supposedly harmful saturated fat than ever but heart disease, cancer, diabetes and obesity are on the increase. This is a 'wellness fail'.

Even when we're on the diets and are exercising we might well be doing the wrong things. These low-fat diets that we used to think were so good for us are actually making us sicker. Doing cardio for long hours each week in an attempt to keep the weight off doesn't work and can actually damage your health. This is a 'wellness fail'.

Travelling the world and questioning what I see in the 'wellness' industry has shown me that there are two things wrong:
1. 'Wellness' is being distorted by the allopathic mindset
2. 'Wellness' has sold out to the supplement and beauty industry

Going for a wellness check with your GP or on a wellness day at work might sound like a good idea. You have some blood taken for testing, maybe a physical examination and you're done: cleared for the next year. The problem is that research shows us that these checks don't make a difference to your health. All they do is give the 'sickcare' system another chance to diagnose you with another condition, prescribe more medication and get you into the system, none of which improves your level of health.

Remember that the tools your allopathic doctor is trained to use are drugs and surgery. Ask them how much they've been taught about the tools of wellness – nutrition, movement and thought. You're in for a shock. Even when medical researchers do try to use the tools of wellness they still use the 'magic bullet' approach. This isn't because they are bad people or stupid. The system educates doctors based on studying diseases and how to treat them. Nowhere in medical school did they study health and how to create it.

Even when allopathic doctors attempt to counsel their patients on lifestyle it doesn't improve their health, so either the patients aren't listening or the GPs are telling them to do the wrong thing, or it's a bit of both. Dr. Edward Miller, the dean of the medical school and CEO of the hospital at Johns Hopkins University estimates that only 10% of all the patients that undergo heart bypass surgery will change their lifestyle beyond two years. So in this model even people who have had major surgery on their heart fail to change what got them so sick in the first place!

Alternatives

The world of Complementary and Alternative Medicine (CAM) is not immune to these myths either. If you're seeing your CAM practitioner then you may think you're escaping the 'sickcare' system. While many health care practitioners who provide alternative or holistic care are on the right track, they are still prone to the myths of the 'sickcare' system.

If they are there to help you when you are sick but not to improve your well-being when you're not sick, then they are operating by Myth 1: Not sick = healthy

If they diagnose you with a disease and then give you some form of remedy or suggest you eat certain superfoods or supplements then they are operating by myths 2 and 3 – You are a machine and you are broken. Colds and flu are not caused by a lack of herbal mixtures or remedies. While these may be used in addressing symptoms, they do not address cause.

If the diet and lifestyle advice they offer you is to treat a specific condition or disease or amounts to 'eat less and exercise more', 'eat low fat and whole grains' or to go vegetarian then they are operating by Myth 4 – You are separate from nature

Wellness has sold out

Drive past any hotel or day spa and you'll see they offer 'Wellness'. If you have a look at what they're offering it's simply a massage. That's it! It might be dressed up in fancy terms with exotic names, it might use stones or bamboo or it might claim to detox and de-stress but it's still a massage. Massages can be nice and can be healing but they are hardly a complete wellness solution.

Look in your local chemist and you'll find the wellness section is dominated by rows on rows of bottles and tubs and tubes selling you all manner of supplements, 'superfoods' or wonder pills of some sort. Research indicates that many of these concoctions are useless, expensive urine makers at best and potentially harmful at worst. How many of these have you tried? How many of these have you taken today? Supplementing smartly can hold some value (see the section on supplements in the *Eat Real Food* chapter) but the creators of the vast majority of these pills, lotions and potions have duped us by clever marketing.

In our desire for well-being, we've opened ourselves up to shrewd marketing and simply applied the old allopathic thinking to the problem and have therefore resolved nothing. We're still looking for a 'magic bullet' without addressing the cause.

The problem with our current view on wellness is that we still think of ourselves as broken machines that are separate from nature and if we can cover over our symptoms, we will be healthy.

The solution lies in addressing the core of our health problem: our lifestyle. There are three main pillars to our lifestyle:
1. CHEMICAL FACTORS – the way we eat (and drink)
2. PHYSICAL FACTORS – the way we move
3. MENTAL FACTORS – the way we think (and feel)

Even when we recognise these factors of lifestyle, in the 'sickcare' paradigm our chemical state through nutrition, our physical state through movement or our mental state through thoughts and emotions, we apply the same level of logic that got us here. We split them up and compartmentalise them. People are fat? Well then they need to eat less fat! Not moving much? Then get on a treadmill and go nowhere! Feeling depressed? Then think positive thoughts!

We pigeonhole the problem and think of these things as separate issues. We diet to lose weight, exercise to build muscle (we might even do both) and meditate to lift our moods. But when was the last time you heard of someone embarking on a plan to tackle all three parts at the same time – how they eat, how they moved and how they thought? That's what we've been doing in our lifestyle programs and practice for years and the results are amazing.

But when did we ever begin to believe that all three worked separately? When did we begin to believe that our mental state doesn't affect your chemical or physical state?

In 1920 there was a famous study where WB Canon asked the Harvard Football Team to visualise their next game. As they anticipated the match Canon found that the player's blood sugar levels increased into the diabetic range. They could think themselves into a diabetic state! When was the last time a diabetes specialist helped their client with mental and emotional stress?

By not addressing all three pillars, how you eat, how you move and how you think, you will never achieve vitality.

CASE HISTORY 2:
What are the consequences?

WHEN I practiced in Scotland, a client of mine thought he was doing everything right and, by conventional standards, he was. Rick ate a low-fat diet, flush with whole grains, dairy and supplements. He ran every day for at least an hour and worked out on the machines in the gym twice a week. Rick was trim and fit by mainstream standards and he saw a psychologist semi-regularly to deal with his stress.

Anyone who saw Rick would have classed him as healthy. He had decades of 'healthy living' under his belt, yet he felt that something wasn't right. He was tired most of the time, he had a paunch that he couldn't shift and rings under his eyes. His yearly check-up with his doctor was something he dreaded because, despite all his hard work, his blood tests and blood pressure showed that he was at risk of developing heart disease. Rick's doctor, nutritionist, trainer and psychologist all agreed that he was doing the right things in terms of his lifestyle and that he needed medication to treat his disease.

His test with me showed another picture. His repetitive, one-dimensional training program had caused a lot of damage to his body. His posture slumped when he relaxed his muscles, his nervous system had to work over-time to keep him functioning and the pattern of his heartbeat showed a decreased ability to adapt to stress.

Assessing Rick's lifestyle I noticed that he was eating foods that were labelled heart-healthy but were clearly damaging his gut. He was eating things that he was told by a nutritionist were good for controlling his blood sugar and helping him lose weight but were doing exactly the opposite.

Rick's moods were low most of the time and although he'd seen a psychologist for years, nothing much had changed. It had been suggested he try antidepressants but he resisted. Rick was not happy with his state of health to say the least. He wasn't happy with his physical performance either. Despite all the training he felt like he was going backwards.

If Rick's story here sounds familiar to you, I'm not surprised. This is the picture I see in practice every day. Good people, doing the best they can with the resources their health professionals are giving them, but getting very poor results. What usually happens is that they lose heart, run out of motivation and go back to a 'life of moderation'.

People like Rick put their faith in a system and are being let down. They're doing exactly what their doctors, nutritionists, trainers or therapists tell them to do but don't get the promised results. Health care professionals are only doing what they've been trained to do, following what they believe to be 'best practice', and are essentially doing what their education tells them to do.

Science tells the professional to give the client certain advice and the client does what he is told, but it doesn't work. Who's at fault here? Not the client, they're following the instructions. Not the professionals, they are following the science. Not the scientists, because they are conducting experiments and putting out the results as they are supposed to. So who is it?

Remember, the quality of your questions determines the quality of your answers so if the answers are failing us, could we be asking different questions? Could we be questioning our assumptions?

The result for people like Rick is that even though they started with the best of intentions – to get healthy – they ended up trying to treat diseases. The two approaches are completely different and lead to completely different results.

How did we get here?

No problem can be solved from the same level of consciousness that created it.
ALBERT EINSTEIN

When a couple argues, the joke is that the man wants to solve a issue at hand but doesn't take the time to acknowledge the woman's experience, and the woman is more interested in sharing her experience than solving the problem. The man sees it as a puzzle that needs a solution and it is his role to fix it. He ignores the fact that the situation being presented to him is probably a symptom of a deeper issue and by solving the superficial issue he's robbing his partner of a chance to express herself and work through the underlying problem herself.

We have lived under many myths with regards to our health through the centuries and found many ways of addressing the presenting issues. In early times we used to believe that ill health was caused by demons that invaded and inhabited the body. Only by purging a person of the demon could the illness be cured. Sometimes the person even survived the 'cure'.

We have also believed that illness was caused by 'bad air' or miasma which emanated from rotting organic matter in swamps, bogs and wetlands. The only way to treat and prevent disease was to avoid contact with bad air which, it was believed, came from foul water and emanated from sick persons. Only by avoiding such miasmas could we manage the illness.

Next, we came to believe that sickness came from imbalance in the humors, or from having 'bad blood', and could be treated with bloodletting. This involved using leeches to suck out the bad blood or simply nicking a vein in the arm or neck to let the blood flow into a container.

Next in the line of causes of disease was the germ theory. We believed that diseases were the results of germs invading our body and causing damage which resulted in illness. Sanitation with modern sewer systems offered us ways to avoid many deadly bugs by flushing them away, and when allopathic medicine harnessed ways of killing germs with antibiotics, it did so with astonishing success. No longer was the common cold a deadly disease, now a single course of antibiotics relegated the illness to a mild inconvenience. No longer was an infection life-threatening, it was now a manageable condition.

Antibiotics to treat bacterial infections have created amazing ways of addressing infections in life-threatening situations. With infection controlled and anaesthetics improved, surgery became more effective because more people survived it. Surgery can now be used to repair things like a hole in the heart of an unborn child, which is a truly amazing feat. Victims of trauma, such as car accidents, can be put back together by remarkable people with extraordinary skill.

Unfortunately those tools have been utterly useless in actually getting to the cause of ill-health. Nothing in the arsenal of medicine at this point has been able to make a meaningful dent in the 'ominous tide' of chronic illness that is sweeping the planet.

The scary fact is that the overuse of antibiotics on ourselves and in our food production system, have created antibiotic resistant superbugs that close down entire hospitals and schools when they strike.

> *The world is headed for a post antibiotic era,*
> *in which common infections and minor injuries*
> *which have been treatable for decades can once again kill.*
> DR KEIJI FUKUDA, WHO ASSISTANT DIRECTOR GENERAL FOR HEALTH SECURITY

This antibiotic binge that we've embarked on has also destroyed our microbiome, the cloud of bacteria that live in and around us and are vital to our well-being. Professor Martin Blaser is the director of the New York University Human Microbiome Program and former Chair of the Department of Medicine has some sobering news. Some forms of bacteria that have shaped our evolution over millions of years are under threat of extinction because of current medical practices.

Bacteria, fungi, yeast, viruses and parasites, we've learned to fear these critters, and for good reason. When they are out of balance or go unchecked by our natural defenses then we can be in for some serious infectious diseases. *E. coli* is a type of bacteria that farmers, food producers and kitchens all fear. They could get shut down if this bacterium contaminates their produce. If *E. coli* gets into your system in the wrong place or is out of balance you can get a nasty case of the runs at best and it could even be fatal.

But it might surprise you to learn that in some parts of your body *E coli* can live in balance with the rest of your microbiome. *E coli* can be a normal, productive member of your habitat. It might surprise you to learn that we are now beginning to realise that some of these supposed nasties are only nasty when they are out of balance and are vital to our well-being when *we* are in balance with *them*.

Now we live in a new age where a new myth comes to the fore. We think our genes are making us sick. Now that we have sequenced the human genome and that the price of sequencing the genes of more and more people is becoming cheaper and cheaper, we are arriving at the conclusion that our genes make us sick.

With the knowledge that our genes make us sick we have forecast that drugs can be invented to control or silence the faulty genes and cure the diseases. The problem is that just because we are beginning to learn to decode the instruction manual for life does not mean that we understand it.

Researchers I have interviewed are becoming jaded by the layers of complexity that our genetic code produces. There is a common theme in which we find a new protein or enzyme that promises to be the next big thing in the treatment of cancer, but as we discover more about it we learn that it's not as simple as we thought.

One example is an anti-cancer, tumour suppressing protein called P53. When its gene is damaged and it doesn't work anymore we are much more susceptible to cancer. With this knowledge, cancer researchers have thought boosting levels of P53 might be helpful in treating cancer. The problem is that P53 also plays a role in blocking most chemotherapy combinations. The story is far more complex than we realise.

Again, despite all the headlines you may have read in the media about new 'wonder drugs' that fix broken genes, none of them has lived up to their promise. Even one of the world's most prominent geneticists, J. Craig Venter, expressed his disappointment with our lack of breakthroughs since the human genome was mapped, and called it a 'bust'.

The snag with all of our technological wizardry is that it has not addressed the underlying problem. Like a man solving the superficial issue of his partner without first listening, we have become very good at inventing more refined ways of patching over issues instead of taking the time to truly understand what is being brought to us, and then helping to address the underlying problem.

An unintended outcome of all of these theories we've described here is that they make the patient a passive victim. None of these empower us beyond telling us to stay away from sick people, take pills and that our fate comes down to a genetic lottery.

The problem is that it has now become normal for us to be sick: we've accepted it as an inevitable part of our lives. The fact that 80% of the industrialised world will have at least one chronic, degenerative, incurable disease while they are in their young, active and productive years is *not* normal. It's *average* but not *normal*. We've passively accepted that getting sick is a normal part of life and so have waived our own responsibility for the issue.

We may be living longer thanks to sanitation and a select few medical discoveries but we are, right now, the sickest version of the sickest species on a planet. And guess what? If our genes are to blame, then abandon all hope until our 'magic bullet' drug has been invented. If our genes are to blame then there is nothing we can do about it until someone invents the pill, lotion, potion or procedure to fix us so we might as well carry on doing what we're doing anyway.

Science tells us differently though. Science tells us that your genes do *not* determine your fate. Science tells us that your lifestyle determines your fate and has far more of an effect on your well-being than your genes do.

As the saying goes, "If the only tool you have is a hammer, every problem looks like a nail." We have many good people in the allopathic paradigm doing work that they know to be worthwhile, but they are working in a system designed around the myths of the 'sickcare' system.

     MYTH 1 – Not sick equals healthy
     MYTH 2 – You are a machine
     MYTH 3 – You are inherently broken
     MYTH 4 – You are separate from nature

Even the way we practice wellness doesn't shift our thinking. We're still squashing symptoms in a mechanistic, reductionist way that is artificial, and without regard for our true nature. 'Eat less, exercise more and think positively' is simply not enough.

What do we want to do differently?

If you dig a hole in the ground you'll have a pile of soil lying on the grass next to the hole. The hole, however, is not an actual thing. It is a 'no-thing'. It's the place the soil used to be.

If you block the light of a candle you will cast a shadow on the wall where there was once light. The shadow is not an actual thing. Instead the shadow is a 'no-thing': it's the place the light used to be.

Like the hole in the ground and shadow cast on a wall, sickness and ill-health is therefore a 'no-thing'. It's the absence of health and vitality.

We need to begin to think about health in different terms, to change our mind, to change our paradigm. Right now sickness is a 'thing' that doctors are taught to diagnose and treat. My university lecturer in systemic pathology (the study of diseases) told us to imagine a disease as a solid object. It was a useful concept when trying to memorise the many diseases we had to know about, but it's a way of thinking that isn't helping us to get healthy.

The entire 'sickcare' system is built on this idea, that sickness is a thing that needs fixing instead of a lack of health that needs to be created.

What we could be doing is asking different questions. The questions we have been asking are:
- How do I cure symptoms?
- How do I temporarily mask the problem?
- How do I get to feel 'ok' as soon as possible?
- How do I treat disease?

Questions that would be more useful to ask:
- What is my vision for my life?
- How do I live a bigger life?
- What is vitality?
- Where does vitality come from?
- How do we create vitality?

To answer these questions you have to begin to see yourself in a new light, and begin to view your vitality in new ways. You then begin to find new answers, to see new possibilities and to transcend old limitations in new and exciting ways.

Let's review the myths of the sickcare system and see if we can find new assumptions to give us some insights.

Current Beliefs	Vitalistic Beliefs
Not sick equals healthy	Optimal function equals healthy
You are a machine	You are an ecosystem
You are separate from nature	You are an animal
You are inherently broken	You are innately intelligent

What if we don't change?

The price of staying the same is high. How high, you ask? Well, how high can you count?!

As individuals, every day we choose to keep operating by our old assumptions and old ideas we sacrifice our own human potential. We are following the advice given to us by the powers that be and it's not working. We are sicker than we have ever been. We might be existing for longer but I would question whether we are truly living and inspired.

Epigenetics is the fascinating study of how we can actually change the expression of our genes and pass this on to our children as our parents, grandparents and recent ancestors did for us. We are affected by what they ate, drank and smoked. We are affected by how they moved. We are affected by what they thought and felt and our children and grandchildren will be similarly affected by us.

Several remarkable experiments have suggested that any animal forced into a lifestyle that is inappropriate to their biological makeup suffers health problems. In animal studies, these health problems mirror our own health issues in unsettling ways. Over consecutive generations of incarceration with poor nutrition, movement and mental stimulation animals become depressed, show poor socialisation and aggression; they become obese, lose the ability to reproduce; their skeletal structure weakens and their skulls shrink; they develop major dental problems; and they begin to develop chronic diseases such as heart disease, arthritis, cancer and dementia. Each generation thereafter becomes sicker and sicker.

I believe that we are in the process of doing exactly the same thing to ourselves. We are in a zoo of our own making, a self-imposed societal cage that is not only robbing us of our potential but also making us sick in slow motion. Like slowly turning up the temperature on the proverbial frog we have hardly noticed the change until it's too late.

The good news is that the changes are reversible up to a point. We can stem the tide, we can stop the slide. To do this we have to act and we have to take responsibility for ourselves and our destiny.

What if we do?

We live in an exciting time where our technology offers us new ways to experience the world. New ideas and technologies can help us live longer, to give more, create more and serve more.

We also live in a time where we have learned and developed creative ways to kill each other and drive our species off the map. From war and conflict to poverty and climate change, we have invented myriad ways to induce pain and suffering in others and in ourselves. While this is a much larger societal problem, I believe the solution lies with each and every one of us.

Put this together with the impending reality of poor health, reduced productivity and its economic consequences that we've laid out, and we are looking at a bleak picture worthy of a post apocalyptic scene in an action movie. We are in real danger of causing irreversible damage to ourselves and the ecosystems we live in.

We can't look to governments to make the change. The solution will not come from the top down. The problem has come about because that's exactly what we have been doing: allowing the powers of authority to dictate the way we should live our lives.

To turn this situation around we each need to take responsibility for our own lives. We need to invest in ourselves. No one is going to save you. If we can begin to realise our potential by valuing our own lives enough, and begin to be the change we want to see in the world, then we have a chance at a bright future. We have to start with our own lives before we can expect others to change. ●

> *Health is more than a disease-free interlude.*
> *To be healthy is a body toned to maximum performance potential,*
> *a clear mind exploding with wonder and curiosity*
> *and a spirit at peace with the world.*
> PATCH ADAMS

3

You are an ecosystem: from disintegrated machine to integrated ecosystem

Descartes folly: The Mind and the Body.

Calories don't matter.

The victim is created.

Epigenetics: Your genes in conversation.

Follow the dung and save yourself.

You are like a fridge.

Stress can heal.

What really kills you.

$1 + 1 = 5$

Your true nature.

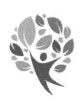

How do we currently view ourselves?

During the Age of Enlightenment, which began in the late 1500s, because of political tension between early scientists and the church in Europe, the naturalists, as they were then called, developed the mind-body split also know as Cartesian dualism. To appease the all-powerful church, which believed that the mind and the soul were their holy domain, the enlightenment scientists claimed knowledge of the body only and left the mind and spirit to the church. By focussing only on the body they weren't challenging the church's authority and would be allowed to continue their learning unimpeded.

This Cartesian way of thinking – the separation of mind and body – led us to understand more and more about the basic building blocks of the universe, allowing us to manipulate nature to create new chemicals that have changed the world, split the atom, sent man to the moon and produced computers and machines that have improved our lives.

This way of thinking has been useful, through it we discovered breakthroughs in our understanding of the world. During this time Isaac Newton developed the 3 physical laws of motion and the laws of gravitation which were a stunning breakthrough in science and opened up our understanding of the universe.

Our mastery of nature seemed to be absolute as we harnessed new technologies, kick-starting the industrial revolution. This era saw the rise of steam power to run gigantic machines and we began to understand how to manipulate metals, chemicals and fabrics. Farming became more productive and gas lighting came into being.

Clearly the process of breaking things down into their constituent parts to understand the whole – called reductionism – has been immensely useful in our technological progress. By understanding the different moving parts of something we have gained a better understanding of how it works and how we can fix some problems. If a watch breaks and we know what the different parts do, then we can find the broken one and mend it or replace it. Thanks to our technological innovation, we can even do this on a microscopic scale.

But, it has also led us to think that we are machines, that we are purely mechanical, like the steam engine. When one part of the machine goes wrong, we simply modify that part and it will be fixed and up and running again. When we apply this same thinking to the human body it allows us to understand one dimension of how the body works and how to fix some things, like accidents and trauma. If you're in a car accident and your leg is badly broken you're fortunate enough to have a good orthopaedic surgeon to set the bone, a vascular surgeon to fix the arteries and veins and a plastic surgeon to give you a skin graft.

Similarly, thinking of the heart as a pump is useful in mechanically replacing or repairing a heart or one of its valves. The very first heart transplant happened in Cape Town and the pioneering surgeon, Dr Chris Barnard famously said, "the heart is just a pump."

This thinking has some limitations though. Some of the most common procedures performed to unblock the arteries of the heart are ineffectual in improving health. Common procedures for heart disease, called angioplasties and stents, do not prolong life in stable individuals. Heart bypass surgery itself prolongs life in less than 2-3% of patients who receive it.

The problem is that we now see that the reductionist mindset that led to these miracles of modern medicine does not address the cause of the greater problem: they are only a temporary patch and not a solution. By thinking of ourselves as machines we have separated ourselves from nature and not only damaged our own well-being but that of the entire planet as well.

The health problems we face are now chronic and degenerative in nature. They are the result of years of damage inflicted on our bodies and to heal that damage we need a different way of thinking.

Breaking things up into ever smaller parts in order to understand them is a reasonable way to begin to understand something, but putting them back together to grasp how everything works in unison is much harder and usually comes later in the development of science. In fact you could call this an art, not a science and that is a direct contradiction of the allopathic system.

To grapple with many of our current global challenges, especially health, we need to begin to put the pieces back together and this is not a new concept. Modern medicine has motivated such change over the last few decades. Even with the rise of Complimentary and Alternative Medicine (CAM) and Chiropractic, whose strength lies in the fact that they try to see a patient as a whole person, only a minority of allopathic medical practitioners are taking note.

How does this shape our thinking?

Compartmentalised in space

Modern research clearly shows that your mind and body cannot be regarded as two distinct and separate units. They are inseparable: it's your mind-body. A simple example of this is the placebo effect. When someone believes they are being given a drug that will heal them but the drug is really a sugar pill, their belief triggers self-healing capacities that can be more powerful than any drug we have invented. This is a process that most researchers discount instead of harness.

We know that your thoughts and feelings create a cocktail of chemicals in your body that can either create health or cause disease. Your mental and emotional state can literally switch genes on or off and affect your hormones, your energy levels, how you digest food, how your heart works, how you fight infection and anything in between.

The heart is far more than a pump. It's a neuroendocrine gland and also an epicentre of nerve activity that influences your physiology and creates an electromagnetic field that extends beyond your own body to influence those around you.

We are realising that we are far more than just biochemical machines. We are complex ecosystems. Unfortunately this revelation has yet to reveal itself in the day to day practice of 'sickcare', where you as a whole person, a mind-body, are not considered.

Our current belief is that we are made up of individual parts and that only by understanding the individual parts can we better understand the way the whole mind-body works. You go to one doctor for your sinus problem and another for a digestive problem and another for depression, never seeing how the three may be linked.

What we're discovering is that allergies are linked to what happens in our gut, and what happens in our gut has a strong influence on our state of mind. It doesn't stop there, though: we also know that our state of mind has a massive impact on our immune system, too! Our mind-body is far more integrated than we ever imagined.

44

Compartmentalised in time

Just as reductionist thinking stops us from integrating our mind-body right now, it also stops us from realising that where we are a product of where we've been before – our journey.

We tend to ignore what the past might mean for our health right now. Here in South Africa I often get big men who come into my rooms with pain of some sort. James was a particularly large ex-rugby player who had back pain. He told me it started after he bent over to pick up a pencil. When I asked what else might have contributed to the issue he didn't think his previous 20 years of being battered a few times a week on the rugby field could have contributed. He said, "It's been 10 years since I was forced to stop playing because of my hip injury."

James was in the front row of the scrum (a very physical position involving two sets of 8 men locking heads and pushing against each other) week after week for 20 years and had suffered many back injuries. Because they happened more than 10 years ago, he felt they didn't have any bearing on the present. "It is only my knees and my ankle that are still injured."

Here is a very smart man, who is so steeped in the idea that he is like a machine, but he is unable to make the connection between what he's put his body through in the past and how it's affecting him in the present.

James, like many others, came to realise that he is now paying the price for previous stressors to his mind-body. This empowers him to take control of his circumstances and not only help his mind-body heal but also to optimise well-being and achieve his human potential.

James would have been quite unaware that the damage that took years to happen will take months to repair. If James had not realised how long this damage had taken to accumulate and the types of stressors he had been exposed to, he would not have realised that the pencil was just the last straw.

In James' mindset a painkiller or quick fix to remove the immediate pain would solve the problem and allow him to continue his life. He was unaware that this would set him up for recurrences of the problem and make him susceptible to other health troubles. That mindset would be the path to irreversible damage.

When I see people who have signs of this permanent damage to their mind-body they all say the same thing: "Why did none of the other doctors tell me this?!" When I hear those words I feel the responsibility of a system that has failed us.

If we believe that our state of health is random then we are passive victims to our circumstances. If we are victims then there is very little we can do to prevent health problems like sickness and pain; we are then dependent on some authority to fix us, like a car needs a mechanic to fix it.

Compartmentalised in cause

When you view yourself as a machine that is separate from nature and inherently broken, it makes sense to look for a simple linear cause and effect relationship. We want to find what single thing causes a condition of disease so we can make sense of the world and move on.

A great example is: smoking causes lung cancer. This is what we hear all the time: it's trumpeted from the roof tops and it's true enough but it's not completely true. Life is more complicated than that. You see, if smoking did *cause* lung cancer, $X = Y$, then *everyone* who smoked would get lung cancer. But since you're a not a machine it's not that simple. I absolutely agree that smoking causes damage on the cellular level and contains many cancer promoting compounds that raise your risk of cancer by about 25 times. I also agree that the damage smoking does affects your whole mind-body and weakens your entire ecosystem while robbing you of your life's potential. It's not as simple as $X = Y$.

Another mindset is that all the calories we eat are created equally and those burned off are also equal, therefore weight-loss is as simple as calories in vs. calories out, $X = Y$, or eat less and exercise more. When I encounter people who have been sold this idea by the 'sickcare' system, they feel let down because they have gone through periods of starving themselves with mediocre – if any – results. I've worked with people who religiously weigh and measure their food, religiously exercise and still don't seem to be able to shed the weight. I also know of people who can move onto a diet and consume more calories than they normally would and still lose weight.

When we think like this we don't give enough concern to the quality of calories and their ingredients that we are consuming. 100 calories of fresh, organic tomatoes is not the same as 100 calories of hormone and pesticide laden, irradiated and preserved tomatoes. Calories do matter, just not in the way you've been led to believe.

CASE HISTORY 3:
Accumulating solutions

ONE OF MY private coaching clients was a devout dieter but couldn't seem to make any progress. She'd stuck to one diet for many months before trying another, still with no success. She then added exercise to her regime still with no significant weight loss. We addressed not how much food she was eating but the quality of the food; not how much movement she was doing but the quality of movement. These changes started to help her to see some changes, but it was still not enough.

We also looked at her mental and emotional stressors and found she had many deep-seated issues that were affecting her state of mind. Dealing with these issues she began to get drastic results. Only by decompartmentalising her stressors and working on all of them did we make a breakthrough and achieve transformation.

What is the result?

Victim

If we consider ourselves to be machines, at the mercy of bad luck, bad germs or bad genes, then the 'sickcare' system makes complete sense. Waiting for something to 'break' inside us – as it inevitably will – sounds rational. Needing some outside agent like drugs or surgery to fix us seems normal. Being a victim and needing a rescuer in the form of a health authority to cure us is common sense.

As machines we are passive recipients for treatment when things go wrong. Sure we can look after ourselves a little but we have no real control. As machines we're disempowered and reliant on the gifts and skills of the 'sickcare' system to fix us.

In psychology this is called 'victim mentality' and it's not a good way to progress through life if you really want to thrive and not just survive. Being a victim means that you have no control over your own well-being; you have no say over your own destiny; you're always searching outside of yourself for your next fix, and you're at the mercy of anyone who says they can save you.

Linear thinking

If you have a headache you assume that something has broken so you take a pill that finds its way to the fault and shuts it down. If we have high cholesterol then we take a drug that goes to the liver and stops it from producing so much cholesterol: problem solved. If you have high blood sugar then it's a fault in your body that needs a drug to fix it and once the blood sugar is lowered then the problem is solved and you're back on track. If you have depression then you have a problem with the production of your 'happy' chemicals and taking medication that boosts these chemicals will solve the problem.

Simply put: machine broken, drug taken, machine fixed.

That level of thinking creates exactly the situation we are in now. We are the sickest version of the sickest species on a planet we are making very sick. No one is coming to save you.

Lowering cholesterol does not mean that the problem is solved, it's just covered over. In fact, lowering cholesterol with drugs has very questionable benefits, negates some of the fitness effects of exercise and has been linked to a whole host of other problems from diabetes to chronic pain to cancers.

Aggressive lowering of blood sugar with drugs in diabetics can actually cause death. Using antidepressants affects the whole range of human emotion, positive and negative, dulling your experience of life. In reality these drug work about as well as a placebo (sugar pills) and they don't contribute to long term change for most people and actually make 1 in 4 people worse. Amazingly in children and adolescents the use of antidepressants doubles the risk of suicidal thoughts and agression.

When we take medication like statins to lower cholesterol, a statin doesn't go *only* to the liver, it goes everywhere and affects many things. The same goes for blood sugar lowering, antidepressant and even pain medication. There are no 'side effects' of medication, just effects. Sometimes these are useful and sometimes they aren't but they are always 'system wide', meaning that they affect *everything* not just the one faulty part of your body.

Ecosystems are so complex that causation can work both ways. For instance, in Naseem Taleb's book Antifragile he gives us the following example: we think that

48

our bones get weaker and more brittle because we get older. Research in the Journal *Nature* has shown that it can also work the other way: loss of integrity and health of the bones can cause ageing and, in men, fertility and sexual function problems, too.

In the gym I see many people treating their bodies like machines. They isolate and work separate body parts like abs, biceps, quads and chest in very limited and disconnected ways. When you treat your body like that you develop imbalances and dysfunction that lead to defence and decay and injuries are the inevitable result.

What am I?

The truth is that you are not a machine. As useful as that metaphor has been, it is time to move on. It is time to recognise yourself as more than a machine or reducible to the sum of your parts. It is time to recognise yourself as an ecosystem.

You are not an individual sitting reading this book. You are an ecosystem of some 75 trillion cells. In fact, by sheer number, you are more bacteria than human because there are 10 times more bacterial cells in and on your body: you are an ecosystem.

Each of your cells is the powerhouse of your life. Each of them has the same functions that you have. They have a way of taking in, digesting and using nutrients just like you do. They have a way of liberating energy to use just like you do. They have a way of fighting infection. They are a communication and processing system and much more – just like you are.

Each of your cells has exactly the same genetic code. A cell from your heart has the same genetic code as a cell from your brain or a cell from your big toe. The difference between them is how that genetic code is expressed: which parts are turned on and which parts are turned off. This is called epigenetics.

Your experience of life in your mind-body is the sum total of all of those cells working together. The cells work together as individual organs, the organs work together as systems and the systems all work together as your body.

We know that a forest is an ecosystem and the health of the whole forest depends on the health of each individual tree. Since you are an ecosystem, too, your health depends on the health of each individual cell in your body.

Take one of your cells and put it in a petri dish in a lab and give it the nutrients it requires and it will continue to grow and thrive. Put that same cell in another dish that contains toxins and it will go into defence mode instantly. Leave it there and watch as defence mode is overcome causing decay, degeneration and eventually, cell death.

If we save the cell before it dies and we put it in the dish with the nutrients, we would see that cell begin to repair itself as much as possible. What we see is that your cells can be in only one of two states: growth and repair or defence and decay, there is no in between.

This is exactly what cellular biologist, Dr Bruce Lipton, discovered in his laboratory experiments in the 1960s. Realising the states of cell growth and defence, Lipton took this experiment one step further and used stem cells. Stem cells have the ability to turn into any kind of cell, be it an eye or a heart, a liver or a big toe cell. You could say that stem cells have not decided what they want to be when they grow up. The key to Lipton's research is that each of the stem cells was genetically identical.

Lipton placed the genetically identical stem cells into 3 separate dishes each with different environments. In dish A the cells formed muscle cells, in dish B they formed bone and in dish C they formed fat cells. What's remarkable here is that these cells were genetically identical, yet they responded to different environments and formed different types of tissues accordingly.

This simple experiment contradicts what has been taught in university until very recently and is a departure from the claims of the popular press that our genes are responsible for our ills. This is called genetic determinism. When you hear on the news that science has found a gene for cancer, or shyness or obesity, they are referring to genetic determinism and that's old science. Any health professional taught in the 'sickcare' model is taught that our genes control our biology.

Lipton's elegant test actually shows that the environment shapes the expression of our genes. He says that humans are like skin covered petri dishes and that our environment is like the environment of the petri dish. What we've realised is that our environment determines how our genes act just as the environment in the petri dish controlled the fate of the stem cells. Our environment determines which genes are turned on and which are turned off, which are expressed and which aren't.

Our environment is made up of three elements:
- CHEMICAL – what we eat and drink, the drugs we take, the cosmetic products we put on our body and chemicals in our food, air and water.
- PHYSICAL – accidents, injuries, how we move, sit, stand and sleep. Electromagnetic radiation from sources like cellphones and WiFi.
- MENTAL – Our thoughts, beliefs, perception of events and how they affect us.

This is the study of epigenetics; it's revolutionising our understanding of ourselves, the world around us and our place in it. There is another famous experiment that beautifully demonstrates the power our environment has on the expression of our genes.

Randy Jirtle and Jennifer Weidman from Duke University in North Carolina, USA, found that an 'enriched environment' can overrule genetic mutations. Agouti mice are useful in laboratory research because they are prone to becoming obese and developing cancer, diabetes and heart disease because of a genetic mutation. That mutation also gives them their characteristic yellow coat.

In the experiment, female mice were split into two groups: one group received food enriched with folic acid, vitamin B12, betaine and choline while the second group had standard mouse food. The groups ate their different food before and during pregnancy and the pups that were born were very different.

The pups born to mice fed the enriched diet were lean, brown and very healthy compared to the fat, yellow and sickly pups born from the other group. The striking thing about this result is that the two groups of mice were genetically identical.

Epigenetics tells us that genes are not set in stone: their activity can be switched on or off. This switching happens when something in a cell's environment triggers one of those switches. When Dr Lipton put a stem cell in a petri dish that had the triggers for bone formation, the cells turned into bone. When the environment triggered muscle the cell became muscle. Both cells were genetically identical but the environment triggered different reactions. The agouti mice were also genetically identical yet the difference in the food they ate meant that their babies were drastically different.

Our environmental triggers, these chemical, mental and physical factors are the things that then activate or deactivate our genes. As Dr Lipton says, "Our genes load the gun, but environment pulls the trigger."

By studying human twins we find that genes only account for 0-10% of your chance of getting cancer. That means that cancer is very rarely truly genetic in origin and is 90-100% caused by our lifestyle and how that affects our genes.

What this means for us is that the three environmental factors that affect our development (chemical, physical and mental) are the things that will determine how we express health or how we develop disease.

We don't assess our chemical, physical and mental factors every day, but let's use simple terms that we can apply to your daily life.

ENVIRONMENT
        CHEMICAL   = Eat
        PHYSICAL   = Move
        MENTAL   = Think

If we use combinations of those three pillars we can also tease out 3 other key lifestyle factors:
- REST: How we rest, sleep and recover
- NATURE: How we expose ourselves to nature's stimuli
- BREATH: How we manage our respiration

Growth vs Defence
If you take a leaf out of the book of the agouti mice and choose to live in an enriched environment, you will trigger a state of ease, high function, growth and repair in the ecosystem that is your mind-body. In a state of growth and repair your body will be happy to build muscle, shed fat, boost energy, have sharp mental function, be physically strong and flexible, and allow you to make and raise healthy children. In a state of growth and repair your mind-body will move toward a state of vitality and give you everything you need to realise your human potential and maximise your personal performance.

If, instead, you choose to live in a deprived or toxic environment you will force your mind-body into a state of dis-ease, dysfunction and defence. You can be in varying degrees of defence from minor, where you're off your best but not too bad, to major, where you:
- accumulate fat
- cannibalise muscle

- shred areteries
- shrink the brain
- demineralise bone
- imbalance hormones
- distress your gut
- irritate your skin.

You feel drained of energy; you're injury prone and have poor mobility; you experience brain fog and your focus is fuzzy; your libido is low while fertility is compromised and women can have painful cycles, PCOS and endometriosis; and men might suffer from erectile dysfunction.

Defence and dis-ease lead to decay and eventually to disease like cancer, heart disease, diabetes, obesity, depression, anxiety, osteoarthritis, arthritis, chronic pain, MS, thyroid disorders, IBS, chrohn's disease and many more.

In fact many doctors and researchers now consider the chemicals that go along with the defence and decay state, called 'chronic inflammation' to be a 'unified theory of chronic disease.'

Chronic inflammation is associated every chronic disease studied from depression to cancer. Think of it like the trouble maker in a class room that gets other kids to misbehave. The other kid get's caught and the troublemaker is free to continue their mischief.

Chronic inflammation accelerates that rate of ageing of a cell and causes them to breakdown and decay. It moves them from vitality to disease and death. It pays to minimise chronic inflammation by limiting the stressors your mind-body can't resist.

Epigenetics in real life

What all of this really means is that your genes are in a conversation with your environment every second of every day. Every physical, chemical or mental trigger causes a reaction on a cellular level. Your genes are constantly responding and adapting to what you eat and drink, how you move and how you think and feel.

Feed your genes nutrients and they will trigger states of growth and repair that lead you to vitality. Feed them stressors and they will trigger states of defence, decay and disease.

> *We think of our bodies as stable biological structures that live in the world but are fundamentally separate from it ... but that we're far more fluid than we realise, and the world passes through us.*
> STEVEN COLE PHD

The magnitude of the importance of this discovery cannot be emphasised enough. When you go out and exercise, up to 60% of the expression of your genetic code is affected in response to that movement.

Dr Dean Ornish, a medical doctor and researcher writes in Newsweek, "Research shows that improved diet, meditation and other non-medical interventions can actually 'turn off' the disease-promoting process in men with prostate cancer ... My colleagues and I published the first study showing that improved nutrition, stress management techniques, walking, and psychosocial support actually changed the expression of over 500 genes in men with early-stage prostate cancer."

Foods you eat and things you drink will cause changes in how your genes are expressed. Every thought, feeling or emotion, every fight, laugh and cry that you have had or will ever have is reflected in the expression of your genes. Your sleep patterns, what you smoke, the environmental pollution you're exposed and the alcohol you drink have all been shown to change your epigenetic patterns.

We even know that some of these changes survive through generations, that how you eat, move and think will have an effect on your children and their children.

Holism

Alan Savory is an environmentalist who has worked mainly in southern Africa for over 4 decades. He was involved in working to prevent desertification, where lush grasslands were being changed into sandy deserts. In his famous TED talk he relays how they initially thought that overgrazing of elephants was the main cause of desertification. With this in mind they culled thousands of the giant beasts and other grazers to ease the effect on the land.

What happened, however, was exactly the opposite. The desertification continued and even worsened. This is a classic example of how we think we know better than nature and we arrogantly interfere and do more harm than good.

Ecosystems, whether on a mountainside, in a tidal pool, or the ecosystem that is you, are subject to the concept of holism. What this means is that each one is 'whole' and made up of different parts. 'Wholes' have properties that are not present in their parts and are not reducible to the study of their parts. For instance rain forests have the ability to create climates, something which each individual tree in the forest cannot.

Your conscious awareness of this book as you read it is an emergent property of all of your cells put together. Your liver cells cannot be aware of this book, nor could an individual brain cell. Put them all together and consciousness and awareness now emerge like climate control in a rainforest.

Ecosystems are incredibly complex and usually seem to defy the laws of logic because they don't work in a linear fashion. In Yosemite National Park in the USA they reintroduced wolves years after these predators had been wiped out of the area by hunting. This re-introduction was a measure to reduce the number of elk that were eating so many plants and trees that they were causing damage to the ecosystem.

Bring the relatively small number of wolves had some rather interesting effects on the whole ecosystem. Their presence set in place a ripple effect that ended up changing the course of rivers.

The wolves preyed on the elk that then changed their grazing patterns which allowed trees to regrow. The regrowth of the trees stabilised river banks and prevent further erosion. The growth of trees brought back animal life, like beavers, that built dams and shifted the course of streams that affected the course of rivers. This effect is called a trophic cascade.

Ecosystems are also interdependent on the individual species that make them up. The African savannah is made up of many animals and plants and each is dependent on the other in some way. The lion is dependent on the zebra for food; the zebra is dependent on the grass for food; the grass is dependent on the zebra and lion for their droppings and on the remains of a zebra carcass to enrich and fertilise the soil. The lion needs the long grass to hide in so he can hunt the zebra, too. It is an interconnected web: remove one piece of it and you fundamentally alter the web.

No grass? Zebra die of hunger and so do lions because there are fewer zebra and nowhere to hide. No lion? Over population of zebra which overeats the grass, which leads to zebra starvation and then a lack of fertiliser, so erosion destroys the soil and no grass can grown. Each is dependent on the other.

The ecosystem of the savannah is not static; it is continuously in flux, adapting and dynamic. If the number of lions goes up, they eat more zebra, so the number of zebra go down. Now the lions have less food so either they have to move on or they die of starvation. This allows the zebra numbers to increase, but if they go too high they will overgraze the grass and then their food source will become scarce. Now they will either have to move on or die of starvation. When they do migrate, the grass can regenerate which allows the zebra numbers to increase along with the lion population.

This method of checks and balances within a system is called homeostasis, or, the ability to self-regulate a dynamic balance. Every ecosystem has this self-balancing, self-regulating capacity.

Because you are an ecosystem, you too are self-developing and self-regulating. Each cell is constantly working to keep itself balanced so it can perform optimally. Heart cells want to beat rhythmically, kidney cells want to filter blood, stomach cells want to produce the right amount of acid and immune cells want to find and destroy invaders.

All these cells work independently and collectively to keep you in dynamic balance. They regulate your temperature, your heart rate, your internal pH, your blood pressure, and much, much more. If you're sitting in the hot sun and your temperature goes up, you begin to sweat to cool yourself down. If you're working out in the gym, demand for oxygen goes up and so your heart beats faster and you breathe faster, too. If your internal pH goes too low and you become acidic, your body leaches calcium from muscles and bones to buffer the acid and balance your pH again.

This kind of dynamic balancing is going on all the time and is maintained and co-ordinated by your nervous system – your brain, spinal cord and all the nerves in your body. More specifically, it's the autonomic part of your nervous system that is responsible for this dynamic homeostasis. This is the automatic part of the nervous system and one which you have no conscious control of in your everyday life.

Follow nature's blueprint

To restore balance we can look to Alan Savory on his quest to address desertification. Having spent many years culling animals like elephants in an effort to help grasslands regenerate only to see the problem worsen, Alan and his teams were brave enough to realise and own up to their mistake and take a bold step to rectify it. In the TED talk Alan has tears in his eyes and you can see the pain that his past actions are causing him, even though they were brought about through the best of intentions.

What Alan Savory's team began to do was mimic nature and find out how they might regenerate the sandy deserts back into thriving grasslands. One of the solutions they found was to let livestock intensively graze on what grass there was and let them fertilise the ground with their droppings and trample these nutrients into the soil. This was a bold and brave step because it flies in the face of conventional ecology which says they needed fewer grazing animals, not more.

The results couldn't have been more dramatic. Alan's before and after photos show once dry and arid scenes, with only a few brown spindly shrubs, now bursting with green leaves and grass to the point that they are hardly recognisable. By following nature's lead Alan Savory managed to regenerate an entire ecosystem by pulling a few key levers.

Homeostasis

Ecosystems use their self-regulating properties to adapt and evolve over time. Just as there were checks and balances in the savannah, so are there for you as an ecosystem. This process is called homeostasis and it is a dynamic balancing act operating in your body every moment of every day, while you're sleeping, eating, working and even while you're having sex. Don't let the 'stasis' part of homeostasis fool you, though: it's a truly dynamic, constantly moving, flexible and adaptive process that is never static.

A very simple example of homeostasis is a fridge. You set it to a cool 2 degrees Celsius to keep your food chilled, and it makes sure that it pushes out just enough cold air to combat the heat from outside and keep the temperature inside constantly chilly. This is much like the balance between stressors and resistance.

If you're opening and closing the fridge door as you're busy in the kitchen, then some of the cold air will escape and the thermostat will register this as a small rise in temperature. The thermostat will tell the fridge to produce even more cold air until it hits the 2 degree mark again. It will then maintain that level until you next open the fridge door. These are checks and balances, stressors and resistance.

If you leave the fridge door open, you're asking the fridge to do the impossible. There is no way it can keep the food chilled because there is a limit to the amount of cold air it can produce. When the stressors (warm air) overpower the resistance (ability to produce cool air) then the balance (temperature) is thrown off and problems arise. In this case your food will spoil.

Your mind-body is constantly keeping tabs on your temperature, pH, blood pressure, hydration, blood sugar and much more. All of these are controlled within very narrow ranges to make sure that you can maintain internal balance for your cells. Each of your cells is also monitoring its own internal state and keeping that in a fine balance too. When balance is achieved in your mind-body and your cells, then you are in a state of ease, growth and repair.

If the equilibrium is upset by stressors then your mind-body and each cell will be working toward restoring that balance. This is a state of dis-ease, defence or adaptation. If this lasts just a short time, then when homeostasis is restored, there will be little to no permanent damage.

As we described earlier in *The Journey,* your well-being is determined by the balance of stressors you are exposed to and the resistance you have from within. Resistance is the ability of the mind-body to maintain our dynamic cellular balance so that we can be in a state of growth and repair. Growth and repair lead to vitality.

By constantly adapting to their environment, each organism within the ecosystem is giving themselves the best chance of surviving and reproducing which, in the natural world, is first prize. Over many years, through the process of evolution, every plant and animal, every living creature on the planet has adapted to its ideal environment. This process never stops.

Each living thing is constantly working to keep itself in that evolutionary sweet-spot of growth and repair. We'll call the ability to self regulate and adapt 'innate intelligence' or 'resistance'.

58

Your innate intelligence is what allows you to heal stressors like cuts and bruises, to fight infection, to build bone, muscle and cartilage, to deal with toxic food and drink and to recover from mental and emotional traumas.

Like the fridge we have limits to what we can resist. If you cut off my arm I'm not likely to grow a new one though with the right kind of help I could heal over the wound and develop a good stump where my arm used to be.

A mother and daughter came in for an assessment. They had been through a lot. The husband had physically abused the mother for many years. He also abused his daughter, though for a shorter period of time. This story played out in their results. In my practice I often see X-rays of people's spines. When I look at them in profile I should see a signature curve in their spine and good healthy bones and discs (the shock absorbers between the bones).

On the daughter's X-rays I could see some changes in the curvature of the spine, a classic sign of trauma, though the bones were still healthy: this tells me that most of the damage is reversible. On the mother's X-ray, however, not only were there changes in the curvature of the spine, but there was also degeneration of the bones. This is irreversible change.

The mother, because of the years of abuse, had progressed from defence to decay while the daughter was still in defence with little to no sign of decay.

If you accumulate more and more stressors that overpower your body's ability to resist them, then your body can't continue to defend against them: you end up going beyond defence and into decay. Once you're in the decay zone you start developing permanent damage. The longer you allow the imbalance to continue the more severe the damage will be.

This happens in your bones, joints muscles and tendons, but it also happens in your nervous system, immune system, gut and hormonal systems. The more you stress the mind-body, the more it defends. The more it defends the less you experience vitality. The more it defends the more it begins to decay and then you experience conditions and diseases.

What do ecosystems need to thrive?
If you were to take a plant and give it good soil and sunlight but no water, what

would happen? It would wilt and eventually die. What if you gave it water and soil, but no sunlight? The same outcome. And what if you gave it sunlight and water but no soil? The same outcome again. What this shows is that what a plant needs to access growth and repair so it can thrive is soil, sunlight and water. It needs all three in order to survive and thrive. We call these things nutrients and in order for an ecosystem to thrive it has to have sufficient supply of biologically required nutrients.

All ecosystems are the same in this regard: they need certain nutrients, like plants generally need soil, water and sunshine. If they are deficient in one or more nutrients they may be able to survive in defence mode for periods of time but it will be impossible for them to really thrive and grow to their full potential.

Now what if you gave the plant everything it needed and it still didn't thrive? Would you say that soil, water and sunlight were no good for the plant? Of course not, you know that they are biological requirements. Since you've addressed those deficiencies you would need to look for other causes.

What if the soil or water was contaminated, or had toxicities? You could give the plant all the sunshine, water and soil that it needed but if the water was tainted your plant would not thrive. Fix that toxicity and keep addressing any deficiencies and then you will see that plant thrive.

Hormesis

Something interesting happens when we place our mind-body under stress. After the disaster at the Chernobyl Nuclear Power Plant in the Soviet Union in 1986 something amazing was documented. 8600 people were involved in the clean-up project and all were exposed to higher amounts of harmful radiation than normal. With all that radiation they were expected to show higher rates of cancer. In reality they showed *lower* rates of cancer than the general population. The radiation they were exposed to seemed to protect them against cancer and this isn't the only time it was observed. Over 3000 scientific studies demonstrate that exposure to low doses of radiation can be beneficial to living organisms.

What's being observed here is called hormesis and these studies showed that if a living thing was exposed to a low dose of radiation then the cells increased their normally dormant repair processes. These repair processes not only neutralised the effects of the radiation but also prevented other disease processes not related to radiation.

Hormesis also explains why your body gets stronger after it has lifted weights. Lifting weights puts mechanical strain on your structure (bones, joints, ligaments, muscles, tendons and fascia), stimulating their repair mechanisms. As the cells repair, they do more than just neutralise the effects of the workout, they build and grow too.

Roman emperors used to be very wary of assassination and they used the hormetic effect to prevent their untimely death. They used to take in very low doses of poisons on a continuous basis. The repeated exposure to the low dose of the poison actually strengthened their system to the point that their immunes systems became tolerant of those poisons.

Living things thrive under some level of stressors to stimulate their growth and repair mechanisms. The key here is that we need enough stressors to grow and repair but not so much that we only defend and decay. There is a 'Goldilocks Zone'where we don't have too little or too much, but just enough. Good stress that helps us grow is called eu-stress and stress that causes us to decay is dis-stress. For the sake of clarity when I refer to stress here I am referring to dis-stress; eu-stress falls under the category of nutrients.

Our current lifestyle has a significant load of stressors built into it. From pollution to sitting to poor foods to work and relationships, I don't think your mind-body is in danger of being under stressed.

How do you help a sick ecosystem become well?

We now know that if the state of defence becomes chronic, it leads to decay and decay leads to chronic disease and ill-health.

When we look at how ecosystems become ill, it's usually not one single factor that damages them. In high school, my sister was involved in a clean-up project for a local ravine in the suburbs of Johannesburg. The river had borne the brunt of many stressors over time and had slipped into a state of decay. Plants were dying, there were no fish in the river and the animal and insect life was minimal. Those plants and animals that were prevalent were species that were neither indigenous nor biologically appropriate and were causing damage and imbalance in the ecosystem.

Air pollution had affected the mosses that grew on the trees and some birds had migrated elsewhere. Water pollution brought chemicals and trash downstream and this had begun to kill off the plants, which resulted in reduced bird and insect life. Plastic bags, bottles, cans and even old clothing accumulated, blocking parts of the river and choking life out of the biomass.

When my sister and her friends went in to clean up the ravine, they started by collecting the rubbish that was almost constantly floating downstream. This was a good start and the area was noticeably cleaner, but it was not enough to help start the rejuvenation.

Next they began to tackle the foreign plant species, removing them by digging them out at the roots. This took time but paid immediate dividends as the indigenous trees, shrubs and flowers slowly started to come through within days. The girls were amazed at how quickly the revival happened. In areas where the recovery was slow they planted new trees and shrubs to help speed things along.

With the help of local government initiatives, the polluters upstream were being put under pressure and so the water quality began to improve. Measurements showed that there were fewer chemicals being dumped into the river. Plants blossomed once again and animals, birds and insects began to repopulate the ravine. Now that the resistance of the ecosystem was stronger something amazing happened: the natural plant and animal life began to crowd out any remaining invader plant species. Because this ecosystem wasn't fighting a losing war on multiple fronts, it was able to better resist one or another form of stressor.

Even though the air quality wasn't addressed, the mosses on the trees began to grow back. With the improved integration of the ecosystem came improved resilience and resistance to external stressors.

With growth and repair happening in the ravine, the girls couldn't afford to let their guard down. Regular sweeps for trash and water quality tests were done. Teams of them went through to dig out any foreign plants that had managed to take root. The change didn't happen overnight. With their efforts the ravine managed to regenerate itself over the next few years. The girls later won a regional prize for their effort.

It was not just one thing that damaged the ecosystem of the ravine but an accumulation of factors that led to its decay. Air pollution, trash, chemicals in the water and invading plants all built up to create this load of stressors.

When we analyse this stress load we notice that it comes in two forms:
- Toxins in chemicals, trash, air pollution and foreign plants.
- Deficiencies of clean air, clean water and appropriate plant and animal life.

When we look at ourselves as ecosystems we can also see the same two forms of stressors across six dimensions:

	Examples of Toxins	Examples of Deficiencies
Chemical (Eat)	Food additives and preservatives, sugars, seed oils, alcohol, processed foods, smoking, drugs, cosmetic products	Vitamins, minerals, fibres, dehydration
Mental (Think)	Strife in relationships, family, financial, work and school, regret, resentment, anger, frustration, fear	Poor self-esteem, poor sense of value in society, low job satisfaction, few meaningful relationships, no celebration of life
Physical (Move)	Trauma, too much exercise, poor posture, poor movement patterns	Sitting, too little movement, spinal subluxation
Rest and Recovery (Sleep)	Over exercise, excessive exposure to screens, excessive exposure to lighting at night	Lack of sleep, lack of recovery time, lack of holidays
Exposure to Nature (Get Outside)	Too much time indoors, too much harsh noise, too much bright and flashing light, too much TV, sunburn, hypothermia	Not enough time outside, not enough exposure to sunshine, not enough exposure to natural sights, sounds, textures, smells and tastes
Breathe	Short shallow breathing	Lack of full, deep breaths

An ecosystem has the ability to repair, regenerate and rejuvenate itself. It has the innate capacity to do this up to a point, but beyond that point it does need some help.

This is much like your mind-body when you become ill; it's not that you've suddenly switched from healthy to sick, but that you've been sliding down the scale of health over time because of an accumulation of stressors in your life – in the way you eat, move and think.

Just as one or two plastic bags in the river don't seem to make the whole system polluted, one or two stressors don't seem to affect you. We joke about the fact that when we were young we could get away with late nights and lots of partying, but when we hit middle age we seem to be affected more. This is a great way to see how constant exposure to stressors degrades your mind-body and makes it more vulnerable to future traumas.

When I begin to address these three elements with my clients, we start by understanding that where our health is right now is the sum total of our nutrition, movement patterns, thoughts and beliefs over our lifetime. These are either toxins and push us down toward defence, decay and disease, or they are nutrients that stimulate us toward growth, repair and vitality.

In their efforts to keep the ravine regeneration going, my sister and her friends had to make sure that the water purity was constantly checked. They also had to make sure that they planted sufficient new trees and shrubs to enable the interconnected web of the plants, animals, insects, fungi, bacteria and everything else that make up the ecosystem to regenerate and recuperate over time.

Once up and running, the network still needed elements from the outside to sustain it: water in the form of rain, clean air and the cycle of nutrients from ground to living things and back to the ground.

The work to revive the ravine started by addressing one stressor – the rubbish. When that was under control (though not completely eliminated) they moved onto the invader plants. Then the water quality was improved by addressing the upstream polluters. One by one they systematically tackled the elements that caused stress on the ecosystem and they let the solutions accumulate.

If the stressors can be classed as deficiencies and toxicities then the nutrients can be categorised as:

1. Purity in water, air, biologically appropriate plants and animals
2. Sufficiency in all the above.

When we look at ourselves as ecosystems we can also see the same two forms of nutrients:

	Examples of Purity	Examples of Sufficiency
Chemical (Eat)	Unprocessed foods, filtered water	Vitamins and minerals, fibres, hydration
Mental (Think)	Celebration of life, self-esteem, balanced perceptions	Self-esteem, value in society, job satisfaction, meaningful relationships, celebration of life
Physical (Move)	Quality of movement	General movement, moving moderately, moving heavy things, moving fast
Exposure to Nature (Get Outside)	Restorative sleep, time off work, recovery after movement, screen free time	Getting outside, sun exposure, exposure to sights, sounds, smells, textures and tastes of nature
Breathe	Full deep breathing	Habitually practicing deep breathing

I approach the well-being of the people who see me in much the same way: we – the person and I – address one stressor at a time and once we have one solution in place, we apply the next. We break this up into different phases and in each phase there is a different focus.

The first phase addresses the outer-most layer of the problem, to seek a cause and create a stable foundation to build on. In this phase we're creating a healing momentum to counteract the actions of defence and decay we've accumulated.

The second phase is about creating a state of growth and repair in which we deal with the accumulated layers of damage by applying more solutions to tackle poor lifestyle habits. Each person decides how much work they'd like to do with the understanding that the more work they do, the better they will feel.

The third and final phase is the lifestyle phase where the person refines his or her eating, moving and thinking habits to allow the body to remain in a state of growth and repair.

As we go through each of the phases, the person assumes more and more responsibility for their results, becoming equally more empowered by their well-being. They accumulate solutions layering them into their lifestyle and each solution that is added makes their changes more powerful.

1 + 1 = 5

A relative of mine is an organic citrus farmer near Port Elizabeth. He told me about some of the ways he harnesses this summative power on his farm. When he first moved from conventional farming to organic farming he had to repair the decades of damage that the artificial fertilisers, pesticides and herbicides had done to the plants, animals and the soil. Since he could no longer use artificial fertilisers, he had to begin using organic compost to get nutrients into his soil. Initially he would put the compost on and he calculated that less than half of what he put into the soil actually stayed in the soil.

His research found that to help the composting process he needed to have the right bacteria in the soil to begin with. These bacteria would break down the compost and release nutrients into the soil that would allow his oranges to grow even better and faster.

The challenge was that these bacteria would only grow if there were certain minerals in the soil, in a particular balance. He worked hard to get the right balance to promote the growth of the bacteria. A while later he re-measured how much of his fertiliser was going into the soil. From his initial measurement of less than 50% return, once the soil balance was right and the bacteria were present, his return escalated to 120%! Putting the two solutions – the mineral balance and the compost – together had allowed this ecosystem to repair and grow. The return was greater than the sum of the investments.

The same holds very true for your health and well-being. Each solution that you apply acts with what is already working and gives you a result that is greater than

66

each individual change. Add together eating, moving and thinking to your recipe for lifestyle change and you will see the power you can harness to express your full potential.

You, the ecosystem

It's useful to imagine that your health, your personal performance, your fitness, the strength of your immune system and everything else that goes inside you can be described in chemical balances. Your hormonal cycles (yes, guys have cycles too!) are a chemical balance; how much fat you carry is a chemical balance; how you fight infection is a chemical balance; how you digest your food is a chemical balance; and even your energy and clarity of thought is a chemical balance.

The chemicals of life are like music produced by an orchestra. As each instrument produces different notes, so too does each organ in your body produce different chemicals. With all the instruments playing at the same time it's vitally important that they stay in rhythm with balance and harmony to create good music. As each organ, tissue and cell in your body takes its turn to produce the right chemicals at the right time, you'll experience the masterful symphony that is vitality.

If, however, we don't hit the right notes at the right time then the full harmony is lost. Chemical imbalances can be as obvious as when alcohol affects your brain: the symphony will obviously be slurred. It can, however, be subtle like the development of, for example, dementia or cancer that takes decades, where the initial change in harmony may be so slight as that it may seem imperceptible.

Some imbalances may affect the reproductive system while others may affect the digestive system. Some may be easy to find and correct where others can lurk in the shadows and be tough to track down, but in the end they are all chemical imbalances of some sort.

The key to having an orchestra that produces gorgeous music that stirs your emotions is the conductor. The conductor is the one bringing all the skill, talent and mastery of each musician as they play their instruments into a balance of rhythm and harmony. The conductor helps each player to come in at the right time, with the right tone, pitch and speed, to play the piece as it was written.

The symphony might survive one musician's mistake or failure, but the failure of the conductor is catastrophic. Not every problem in the symphony is the conductor's fault, but without him there is no chance of the assembled musicians producing wonderful music.

If musical instruments are like the tissues, cells and organs of your body and the music they produce are your chemicals of life, then the conductor is your nervous system. Out in front, just like the conductor, your brain is where virtually every bit of information inside and outside of you is sent and processed. The conductor uses movements of their arms to communicate instructions to the orchestra and your nervous system uses the nerves that run from your brain to each part of your body to send its signals to each cell in your body.

Your nervous system and its lines of communication are so important to your health that, during development of a foetus inside the womb, the brain, spinal cord and nerves begin to develop before any other organ, and every other organ actually develops at the end of each nerve. This design ensures that your master co-ordinating system has direct lines of communication to every other system you possess from the very beginning of your life.

Now, as you keep growing and developing your body needs to protect your nervous system, so your brain becomes encased in the bones of the skull and the spine gets protected by the bones of the spine – 24 mobile bones and 5 fused or immobile bones. This gives you not only protection but also flexibility so that you can grow up bending and twisting, rolling and jumping.

For you to be able to produce the harmonies, melodies and gorgeous sounds your body orchestra is capable of creating, your nervous system must be free of interference so that it can function freely and messages can pass from your brain to your body and from your body to your brain. Your brain and your body must be integrated.

This two-way street is so important that your symphony of health and well-being is dependent on it. You know how powerfully the brain affects the body but you might not know how powerfully the body affects the brain. Nobel Prize winner for his research into the brain, Rodger Sperry PhD said that stimulation coming from movement of the body (called proprioception) is a vital nutrient for the brain – it's as important as oxygen.

68

The brain is powered and balanced by the movement of your body. Movement of your body (especially your spine) acts like a turbine, generating energy that goes directly to the part of your brain that controls homeostasis, that dynamic balance happening inside each of your 75 trillion cells every second of every day.

If integration and full function of the brain and body is necessary for full expression of health, then any interference to the nervous system must necessarily lead to some form of dysfunction, which leads to a state of dis-ease and physiological defence. Remember the effects of a prolonged state of defence:

- accumulate fat
- cannibalise muscle
- shred arteries
- shrink the brain
- demineralise bone
- imbalance hormones
- distress your gut
- irritate your skin.

Left unchecked,
defence and dis-ease leads to decay and
decay leads disease.

> *For those who are awake the cosmos is one and common,*
> *but those who sleep turn away each into a private world.*
> HERACLITUS

4

You are innately intelligent

Your body gives tough love.

Health = Light?

How ageing happens.

What really kills you.

The value of pain.

Your innate intelligence.

What is health?

Health and disease: two sides of the same coin

In May of 2013 four American tourists in Iceland were having a picnic on the ice at the edge of Fjallsárlón glacial lagoon. They had tables and chairs set up for a relaxing meal. Their tranquillity turned to fear when the area of ice they had chosen broke away from the glacier and became an iceberg, floating adrift out to sea.

Suppose you were on an iceberg just outside the arctic circle without protective gear. Beyond feeling the obvious chilliness let's explore how your body handles low temperatures.

Because it's cold on an iceberg and the threat of dying of hypothermia is very real, your intelligent mind-body will go into a defensive response and begin to conserve heat. It does this by drawing blood away from your arms and legs and so keeps heat in the core of your body to support the vital organs. This is a defensive strategy, designed to keep you alive and maximise your chances of getting off the iceberg.

If this redirection of blood is strong enough, it can literally suck the blood out of your fingers and toes, giving your skin red and white patches. This is probably not a very pleasant sensation; people usually report that there is itching and pain, like pins and needles in the extreme.

If you haven't been rescued from the iceberg and your fingers and toes are starved of blood for long enough, the tissue will begin to die. This is frostbite: defence has turned to decay. As frostbite sets in it is supposed to be extremely painful until the nerves themselves freeze and stop firing. Now you're talking about permanent damage unless you get immediate help.

None of this is pleasant but it seems to make sense that your mind-body is doing something intelligent to buy you more time and increase your chance of getting off the iceberg and surviving. You are in defence mode, buying survival time, but too much time in defence and you begin to decay.

It would stand to reason that adopting a strategy to deal with a stressful situation that prolongs your life is an intelligent thing to do. It buys you time to get off the iceberg so that you can live. The danger lies in the fact that the longer you force your body into adaptation, the more damage the adaptive process does, eventually resulting in permanent degeneration.

If the frostbite is left long enough, you will lose your fingers, toes or the tip of your nose. If gangrene sets in, then you can lose entire limbs, hopefully not being killed by the infection.

How amazing is it that your innate intelligence will sacrifice your limbs for the sake of keeping you alive longer, giving you a greater chance of survival? All of this happens automatically, without you having to think about it. This same intelligence is what keeps your mind-body ecosystem functioning in perfect balance every second of everyday.

Luckily for our picnickers, their iceberg didn't drift too far and one of the party managed to jump to shore just as the iceberg broke off and went to fetch help. No one lost any body parts because they were only there for a short time and they had protective clothing to keep them warm.

The cost of adaptation
We've explored the idea that you exist as an interconnected ecosystem of cells, all working in a fine balance we call homeostasis, and now we're realising that your mind-body has the innate capacity to adapt to its surroundings to keep that balance in check.

One of the things that your conductor carefully controls is the O_2/CO_2 balance in your blood and tissues. O_2 is breathed in via the lungs and is transported throughout your body by red blood cells and is used to liberate energy. CO_2 is the waste product of O_2 and gets ferried out of your lungs when you exhale. If the concentration of either one of the gasses gets too high or too low, you're in for some trouble.

When a mountain climber attempts to summit Mount Everest they are obviously using a huge amount of energy at extreme altitudes where the air is thinner and with much less oxygen. Using lots of energy creates more CO_2. Now you're bringing in less O_2 but creating more CO_2 – a potentially deadly situation.

Given enough time to adapt, your intelligent mind-body begins to produce more red blood cells so that you can extract more O_2 from every breath you take and make the process more efficient. So even though the air is thinner up there, you are able to adapt to the situation and get the energy you need to climb the mountain.

People who live at high altitudes often have bigger chests with a bigger lung capacity, too. They take in more air per breath and they have more red blood cells so they can carry more O_2 than the average mountain climber. This is why you'll hear stories of porters on the slopes of Kilimanjaro and other mountains carrying very heavy loads quite quickly while tourists struggle simply to carry their own body weight.

Having more red blood cells in your system also makes your blood thicker and therefore harder to pump around your body. This can put extra strain on your heart. Although most people's hearts can accommodate this extra work, in some of us it may cause problems. Again, the adjustment your body makes to compensate for the altered environment is intelligent, but it can have some detrimental effects over long periods of time. It is designed to help you adapt to escape from less than ideal circumstances for a short periods of time but if ignored and left the cost of adaptation accumulates.

Health = Light

In a lecture I attended a few years ago Dr James Chestnut, author of the Wellness and Prevention Paradigm, was helping us to understand the real nature of health and how we might better understand it. The lecture was set up in the ballroom of a London hotel with a projector showing his detailed slides on a screen behind him. One of the participants, a few rows from the front, put up his hand to ask a question and inadvertently cast a shadow onto the screen. His hand blocked the light from the projector just as would happen with a shadow puppet.

I cannot remember what the question was, but Dr Chestnut suddenly stopped and told us that health was like the projector shining light brightly onto a screen, filling every corner with illumination. Dr Chestnut posed the question: if the light from the projector was partially blocked but most of the information on the screen was still visible, would that be the same as the unimpeded, fully lit screen? We all agreed that it wasn't.

Again he asked: if the screen was filled but the light was dimmed and made the information hard to read, would that be the same as the screen fully lit? Again, we all agreed that it wasn't.

74

Let's go back to the definition of health from the World Health Organisation:

Health is a state of complete physical, mental and social well-being and not merely the absence of disease or infirmity.

Just like the fully lit screen, health is a state of optimum function. Anything less is not health. Anything less is a step closer to what we call disease, and disease is the absence of health.

Imagine that each of the 75 trillion cells that make up your mind-body is like a little light bulb, shining as bright as it can. As each cell shines, it is working on growth and repair, giving you energy, focus, strength, balance, stability, creativity and all the resources you need to be the greatest version of you possible. Combine all the little lights and realise that this is the driving force that gives you life, love, energy, drive, focus, and the ability to create.

Add up each of your little cell lights and suddenly you are an integrated beacon of light, expressing your innate potential at the very highest level. This is your normal state, this is what you are capable of, and this is your birth right. All we have to do to access this state is feed our mind-body the resources it needs in purity and sufficiency and address the deficiencies and toxicities that can dim our lights.

What is disease?

Staying with Dr Chestnut's lecture, if your light is impeded or dimmed, you are not experiencing a full projection of health. I realised that illness was the same as the shadow cast on the screen. If you assume that health was the same as the screen filled with the light from the projector, then illness was like the shadow: a lack of light.

This simple demonstration struck me deeply; it resonated with me intuitively, but went against the allopathic paradigm I was taught at university. Like all doctors, I was taught that diseases were entities that need to be treated. We had been taught to think of diseases as tangible things that you could hold in your hands and analyse. Simply put, we think of them as physical objects. Now I was shown a whole new paradigm. Disease isn't an actual entity, just like a shadow isn't anything tangible. A shadow isn't actually a thing – rather it is a no-thing: the darkness of a shadow is only the absence of light, and so illness is actually the absence of health.

Dr Chestnut asked what could cause the light of the projector to be impaired. We agreed that the shadow was caused by something blocking the light and so would obscure the slide, and he pointed out my colleague's hand. Next he asked what would happen if the projector was lacking enough power to light the bulb fully and so project a weaker light onto the screen? Again, we agreed that it would obscure the slide.

There are two things that could cause the shadow. It was either a lack of power or an obstacle between the projection and the screen.

In health the same principle applies. Either we have something that is blocking our full expression of vitality (toxicities) or we are lacking something that our mind-body needs (deficiencies). Either way, these two issues will disrupt our internal homeostasis and impede the full expression of the light that is our vitality and set us on the path of defence and decay to disease.

Each time we encounter a stressor, we ask the mind-body to adapt and that adaptation comes at a cost, it moves us from growth to defence. Each stressor that creates imbalance and dysfunction, forces us to recalibrate and adjust our homeodynamic internal system and dims that light and reduce our level of function.

When stressors accumulate and your mind-body adapts, you can no longer be in a state of growth and repair; instead you are in defence mode. While this is may be useful in the short term, if you are forced to stay in defence mode in the longer term you move toward decay mode, like frostbite which is irreversible.

The sad thing is that we often live in these early states of dysfunction but aren't ware of it. We think that waking up tired, being overweight, having poor attention spans and memory, feeling weak, having fuzzy focus on life, experiencing poor mobility, poor libido, sexual dysfunction or painful cycles are normal things. None of these is normal. Living in these dysfunctional states is average. Normal is living in vitality.

Deficiencies
In school we learned about vitamin deficiencies and the diseases they caused like scurvy for vitamin C and rickets for vitamin D. These are obvious but what about the less obvious ones?

76

A sedentary lifestyle where we spend a lot of time sitting each day creates a deficiency of movement. A life lived without clear values is deficient in purpose. Staying up late each night and having to wake up early creates a deficiency of sleep. Living a life where we only have superficial relationships and feel lonely is a life lived with a deficiency of connection.

Each of these any many more are biological requirements for vitality. You cannot think of your lifestyle as an a la carte menu where we can pick and choose what you do. For lifelong vitality your mind-body requires all of the necessary nutrients.

Toxicities

Clear examples of toxicities in your mind-body include poisons like cyanide or arsenic. These are acute toxins and are capable of killing people even in very small doses.

What is more important to us though is the accumulation of multiple, seemingly innocuous toxins over the course of a lifetime. Each small toxin is a stress that forces your mind-body to adapt and defend, and as you accumulate more stressors you do more and more defence and decay. These are often subtle, though they have devastating cumulative effects.

Let's look at diabetes, the type that develops during our lives where you don't need to inject insulin, called type 2 diabetes. What happens is that you get starch and sugar by eating things like fruits, sweets, bread, pasta and starchy vegetables that break down into blood sugar inside your body. Blood sugar is unstable, so your body tries to pack it away into the cells as quickly as possible using the hormone insulin. Insulin shuttles the blood sugar from the blood stream, into the cells to be stored for later as glycogen or fat.

When a cell has enough stored energy it stops responding to the insulin and takes in less and less blood sugar; we say that the cell has become insulin resistant. Generally your fat cells are the last ones to become resistant and that's why you keep piling on the kilograms. This is smart because the cells of other organs, like your liver or muscles, don't want to store too much glycogen or fat because it interferes with the normal running of the cell, and so they become more resistant to the fat storing message of insulin more quickly.

If you wanted to, you could stockpile firewood at home to use for cooking but at some point, when all the cupboards are full, you don't want the stuff lying around in the kitchen, living room and on your bed because it's a fire risk and would be highly inconvenient! You'd prefer to store it in a shed, out of the way. That's the same as limiting how much sugar you store in a cell as glycogen and creating a fat cell.

Many years ago, before we learned how to farm and there were no supermarkets, we lived as wild, free humans and the only food we had access to was locally sourced by either hunting for meat or gathering plants as food. When it was summer, we had access to sweet, juicy fruits for a limited season. Loaded with sugars, these fruits would have released blood sugar into our system which would have caused our body to pack it away with the help of the hormone insulin. It might have made sense then to take advantage of all that sugar and pack on the fat for winter insulation and fuel if food was scarce. Eventually the cells in your body would have become resistant to insulin with fat cells being the last to do so, allowing you to store energy for the coming winter.

As the season changed to winter there would have been fewer of those sweet foods that could cause our blood sugar to go up and attract higher levels of insulin. Your body would have been given a rest from all the blood sugar, your insulin levels would drop and your sensitivity to the hormone would return to normal, letting us liberate fat to burn for energy. This smart adaptation has allowed you to store fat to survive winter. As a short term measure and in tandem with the cycle of seasons this adaptation helps us and is an intelligent, healthy and natural response.

Today, with the year round availability of sweet and starchy foods, we keep accumulating the fat and have high levels of unstable blood sugar that has nowhere to go other than fat. Over the years, without the seasonal variation in the availability of sugary foods, the accumulated effects of blood sugar and insulin spikes causes you to continue storing fat and hold onto it. It causes damage to your brain, your kidneys, your eyes, your nerves, your heart and a lot more. The year-round-summer taxes our ability to adapt to high intakes of starch and sugar. When your ability to adapt becomes fatigued and overloaded the long term effects hurt you.

The disease we call type 2 diabetes is the result of an intelligent adaptation that has become overloaded by an excess in our diet. Even before we develop full blown diabetes research suggests that we accumulate damage in a near constant state of insulin resistance. The damage can be much less visible but wreaks havoc on your mind-body. Excess starch and sugar is a toxicity that overloads our defensive systems and leads to decay and disease.

Bug or feature

A woman is on the phone to technical support because she thought her computer was malfunctioning.

"Tech support, Jason speaking, how can I help?"

"Hi there, there's a problem with my computer. Every time I try to delete something I get this silly message that asks if I'm sure. Of course I'm sure, I just pressed delete!"

"Ok ma'am, and if you press 'ok' does it delete what you wanted?"

"Yes, but why does it ask me if I'm sure, is it broken?"

"Well ma'am, have you ever accidentally pressed delete and had the message pop up and then been able to say 'no'?"

"Yes, I guess I have."

"Can you see how that feature has been useful in the past?"

"Well, yes, now that I look at it that way."

"The problem you described is actually a feature that helps you."

"Oh, ok. Thanks for explaining that."

When the woman called, she was annoyed by something she thought of as a problem, a 'bug' in the system that needed fixing. In reality she was describing a feature, an inbuilt protection mechanism that, although potentially annoying, was actually helping her avoid the catastrophic loss of data.

Can symptoms be healthy?

Often in my practice, when someone comes in with a runny nose, a cold or some other malady I'll greet them with a big smile and say, "Congratulations, you are expressing health!" More often than not I get a confused or bemused look. They think they are ill but I am telling them that they are healthy. How does that work?

When you get a fever and a runny nose, is the cause a bug or is it your reaction to the bug? By raising your body temperature your mind-body makes it easier for your infection-fighting immune cells to destroy the germs that might be around.

By creating inflammation in the form of streams of mucous you are sending in white blood cells and flushing out the most likely places where germs could get in – your mouth and nose.

Fevers and runny noses are two very simple examples of symptoms that we regard as signs of disease but are really signs of health; signs of your body fighting back. The same principle is true for pain of many sorts: sore throats, coughs and all illnesses in general. Just like frostbite these symptoms might not be pleasant, but they are intelligent!

If this is true, does it really seem such a good idea to take pills that work against your body and stop your body fighting infection by lowering your temperature and drying up the mucous? Antihistamines reduce the inflammation that your body has created in order to bring in your white blood cells. Similarly, paracetamol and aspirin reduce the fever and inflammation that your immune system has created for the same purpose.

How do you treat disease?

Many years ago, Mother Teresa was asked to join an anti war protest. It was supposed to be a high profile movement and she would have given it much needed credibility and publicity. It was meant to bring awareness to the atrocities and human suffering of war. These issues seemed to be perfectly aligned with Mother Teresa's ideals.

To everyone's astonishment Mother Teresa politely declined. Was she not against wars and the horrors they created? How could this saintly figure possibly not be against people killing, maiming and torturing each other?

She gently explained to her audience that to be anti-anything is futile. By focusing on what you don't want, she said that you will bring more energy to it. To be anti-war was to be too narrowly focused and did not fit with her vision of a peaceful future. The modern day saint explained that if someone cared to put on a pro-peace protest, she would gladly join their ranks.

Every November there is an anti-cancer movement called Movember. Men sport moustaches to show support and raise funds for cancer research. Each year I am asked why I don't sport a 'mo' for the month and every year I give the same answer.

I'm not anti-cancer, I'm pro-health. I have dedicated my life to raising awareness of lifestyle factors that create health and so promote our internal resistance to *all* diseases.

Real wellness is not anti-cancer, anti-diabetes, anti-heart disease or anti any other specific disease: that's too narrow a focus. That mindset falls into the reductionist, mechanistic mistakes of the past that have led us to where we are right now.

It is far more powerful to focus on *what you want*, not what you don't want. Real wellness is pro-health.

To create a new awareness we need to think differently. The quality of the questions that you ask yourself is important because it is your questions that drive you toward the answers. "How do I silence this symptom?" Whether it is frostbite, a runny nose and fever, chronic pain, cancer or any other symptom, they are just that: symptoms of a larger problem. They are not the real illness but signs of the underlying issue.

The question "How do I silence this symptom?" has been useful for many issues. Like firemen are useful for putting out fires, in problems like acute infections and severe traumas, attending to the symptoms can save lives. After the house fire is put out there is still a lot of work to do to restore the building, and the same is true for our health. Saving a life with drugs or surgery is not the same as creating health. After the broken bone has set or the infection is cleared, there is still a lot of healing and regeneration to do.

The new wave of health challenges that come from chronic and degenerative diseases calls for new questions because addressing symptoms does not seem to be working.

Patch or fix?
If you were driving your car and the warning light indicated that the vehicle's oil level was low, you would not put a Band-Aid over the light to solve the problem. Ignoring this warning would cause damage to the engine and possibly lead to complete engine failure.

Why do we act in this way with our mind-bodies? When we use a drug or surgery to patch over a symptom we are effectively putting a patch over a warning light our mind-body is creating. Continuing to ignore the warnings over the course of a lifetime allows more and more damage to accumulate which eventually results in a chronic condition of some sort.

Instead of asking the question, "How do I silence this symptom" we can begin to ask, "How do I create health?" This is a fundamentally different question which invites fundamentally different answers. It is a higher level question, demanding higher levels of thinking.

If you were looking at covering symptoms to solve the problem of a shadow on a projector screen, you could bring in a torch to shine on the dark spot. Now you might have illuminated the shadow but you haven't fixed the problem. The torch light is a poor substitute for the real image that was supposed to be displayed on the screen.

Now that the torch light is there, some people may not even notice that part of the slide was missing. They may begin to think that the partially obscured text is normal. We don't realise that we are not experiencing the full picture. Think of the elephant tethered to the stake in the ground in Thailand, unaware of his potential to break free.

Many patients say they are in perfect health but are surprised when simple tests tell them otherwise. One of the tests I use is to check how far a person can turn his or her head and neck. This is a measure of the health of their spine and nervous system.

A mum told me that she was 'just fine' and was only coming to me because her husband insisted. When we did this simple test, she was astonished to realise that the movement of her neck was limited and much worse on one side. What she thought was normal was not normal at all. She thought she was healthy because she didn't have pain.

Her version of 'healthy' was invariably to wake up tired and not refreshed, to have aches and pains she considered normal, including headaches a few times a week and period pain for which she needed painkillers to function properly. She'd had trouble conceiving and undergone IVF treatment. She thought these things were normal because most of the people she knew experienced similar problems. Although this might be average, it's certainly not normal!

Her X-rays showed significant damage to the bones of her spine, damage that had accumulated over decades. She'd never been in an accident and suffered occasionally from a stiff neck which she associated with stress. Whenever this happened she'd either ignore it or take an anti-inflammatory drug and feel better in a day or two.

Over the years this approach had masked an underlying process of decay and degeneration of her spine. It had caused interference to her nervous system and was quite literally pulling on the base of her brain, affecting moods, energy and putting her body into defence mode. The technical word for this process is vertebral subluxation complex.

From an early age we are taught that masking symptoms is the best way to act. What we learn in our youth drives us to internalise the idea that 'not sick equals healthy'. Through our experiences we learn to believe that we are somehow inherently broken and need outside help to fix us. We get a cold and we are given pills to dry up our runny nose. We get the flu and we are given drugs to artificially lower our temperature. We begin to believe that we are machines and that the chemicals we consume can magically locate our broken parts and somehow fix them.

As we have separated ourselves from nature and raised ourselves above it, we have come to believe that we are immune to the repercussions of this silencing. We are surprised and act like victims when we develop health problems later in life, and again search for the easy way out. We silence the symptoms.

We unknowingly sacrifice our human potential for greatness; we forgo our destiny and we trade our God-given right to fully experience awe at the sight of the majesty of the universe we live in because we've traded 'average' for 'normal'.

If the cause of ill health can be tracked to toxicities or deficiencies, does it not make sense to address these issues to improve our health? Remove the blockage and let your full potential shine through.

Turn the process around

Through my years as a wellness practitioner I've been privileged to work with cancer survivors who have shown incredible strength with support from very special doctors and nurses. One person who told me her story seems to represent the typical progression we see in our current 'sick care' system.

CASE HISTORY 4:

SUE WENT to her doctor with a recurrent pain, was briefly checked and given a painkiller. The pain eventually went away and a few months later she returned to the doctor with low energy. Once again a drug was administered, this time a pill to boost low thyroid function, which can cause slumping energy levels, and again she seemed to improve for a while.

Sue returned to the doctor a third time that year with all of her symptoms worse, but now with unexplained weight-loss. This is a sure indicator of a potential 'red flag' and Sue was referred to a specialist for scans which revealed a cancerous tumour. Sue was told she required surgery to remove the tumour, followed by a programme of radiation therapy. When Sue asked her doctors what she could do to improve her health, she was also told that what she ate and how she exercised or dealt with stress would make little difference to her cancer.

Her weight plummeted further, her pain was almost unbearable and she could only sit upright for a few hours a day. After much of the tumour was removed and repeated sessions of radiotherapy, Sue decided to take control of her own health. She began to eat higher quality foods and cut out all the junk. She began to walk every day, even if only a few metres and she discovered meditation as a way to clear her mind and create mental and emotional balance.

With these new measures she began to feel better. Her energy returned, she began to put on weight and her pain affected her less. Next she sought out our help to address her vertebral subluxation and align her spine and nervous system to help her mind-body integrate and move further toward growth and repair.

A few months later her tumour was practically gone and the doctors credited her turn-around to the surgery and radiation therapy. They completely dismissed her notion that her lifestyle changes had anything to do with her improvement. Sue continued with her new lifestyle and felt better than she had in decades.

Sue is a classic example of how our 'sick care' system is set up. First we wait until symptoms start, then we go to a health care provider who is trained in patching symptoms. If this doesn't work we are sent to specialists who can then escalate the degree of symptom patching with more powerful tools. Only after all this fails do people find lifestyle change as a way of improving their own health; it is usually the last step.

I believe that in the new paradigm of wellness a whole new approach to health is emerging. We need to investigate and identify the source of our current persistent symptoms. Instead of having symptoms treated as a first line of attack, we'll proactively work to create purity and sufficiency in our lifestyles first. From a young age we'll learn some of the fundamental principles of our biology: how to eat, move and think in ways that feed our wellness genes and help us express our full potential. We will be taught to take ownership of our mind-body and to revel in the feeling of vitality and all the power it brings.

This will result in far fewer health problems as we'll be more resistant to both chronic conditions and infectious illnesses. This foundational approach would yield results almost immediately as we would begin to tap into our human potential and increase our personal performance as individuals, families and communities.

Only if this fails should we then turn to medication, surgery and the specialists – our fire department on standby for when they are needed. By the time we reach this point we will have improved our well-being so much that, should we require potent drugs or surgery, we would tolerate them much better and recover from them faster. Instead of undergoing rehabilitation only, we would have experienced a successful *pre*habilitation.

This vitalistic approach will turn our current 'sick care' system upside-down and empower people to look after themselves. No one is coming to save us. We are the only ones who can make the changes needed. Medics, Chiropractors, Naturopaths, Homeopaths, trainers, nutritionists and many other health care professionals would act as guides and teachers first and foremost and as therapists second.

You are in charge. No one is coming to save you. Look for guides, not saviours. ●

With full awareness you become aware of this organismic self-regulation; you can let the organism take over without interfering, without interrupting; we can rely on the wisdom of the organism. And the contrast to this is the whole pathology of self-manipulation, environmental control, and so on, which interferes with this subtle organismic self-control.
BRUCE LEE

5

You are an animal

Fish hospitals?
Why medicine hates biology.
The Human Zoo.
Stress that heals and stress that harms.
Obese lions?
The domestication of humans.

The one problem with the word homeostasis is that in Greek it means 'standing at the same level', which seems to talk about the system being static or uniform all the time. But as we've just discussed, what happens in the cold or at high altitudes is anything but static; it's very dynamic. The word homeodynamics is sometimes used to prevent this confusion but there is a better option.

Dr Bruce McKewan of the Rockefeller University is one of the world leading experts on how the body adapts under stressful conditions to maintain its internal balance. He uses the term allostasis, which translates to 'remaining stable by being variable.' We'll deal with that in the next chapter but for now all we need to know is that dynamic balance is the name of the game.

Humans *vs* Animals

> *Nothing in biology makes sense except in the light of evolution.*
> THEODOSIUS DOBZHANSKY

In his book, *The Wellness and Prevention Paradigm*, Dr James Chestnut comments that during the 1970's the polluted shores of the Great Lakes of North America were flooded with thousands of dead and dying fish that boasted grotesque tumours. The birds that fed on these fish also showed signs of illness, laying eggs with brittle shells and losing their bright plumage. Scientists studying the problem were concerned that the fish and the birds native to this specific area may become extinct.

In South Africa we have seen oil spills off our coasts affecting, most notably, our penguin population. This created public sympathy for our sea life and outrage at the spillage. This same situation has been mirrored around the world wherever pollution has been let loose on ecosystems.

In the case of the Great Lakes or South Africa's penguins, do you think that there would have been biologists and zoologists who might have suggested building fish or penguin hospitals and giving fish and penguins drugs while performing fish and penguin surgery while ignoring the pollution? No, that just sounds silly.

What would have happened if the environmentalists suddenly stood up and said that the cause was faulty genes? How would the scientific community respond if it was suggested that this bad DNA had created the cancers that had decimated the food chain, and that the only solution to remedy the problem is to create drugs that target the faulty genes and silence them? Again, this sounds more than a little odd.

But isn't this exactly what we are doing to ourselves? This thought pattern betrays our underlying belief that we are somehow separate, or even above, nature. We seem to think that we are not animals.

My Chiropractic education was modelled on that of a medical doctor for the first three years. While many of my friends were studying medicine and were surprised to find out that our depth of anatomy, physiology, biochemistry, pathology, immunology and other subjects was as deep, if not deeper, than their own, we also had one thing in common. Our study of biology and our place in nature was cursory at best and at worst regarded as a relic of a 'classical education' that had outlived its usefulness. The subject of biology in health care education was just a hurdle to be cleared to move onto the important stuff.

Look at any health care course – from medicine to Chiropractic to nursing to nutrition – and you'll find something quite curious. When we studied health care in a university or college of some sort, our classes and departments are in a separate region on campus from the place where biologists or zoologists studied other animals. Sure, in the first year there might have been some study of mice or frogs in a lab but more and more this is being minimised. Study of health has been moved further and further away from the study of biology.

This might sound like an odd distinction to make, but the study of medicine is a branch of biology which is the study of living things. We know that issues arise when a health care speciality loses sight of the bigger picture and now we realise medicine has lost sight of biology. Humans are primates of the same family as chimpanzees, monkeys and gorillas. We are also mammals of the same group as whales and elephants. We are animals and we've separated ourselves from the animal kingdom and nature's laws.

Evolution is a key principle in the study of life; it's the process of adaptation over many generations that allow living things to adapt and progress. Evolution has taken us from single celled amoebae to complex multi-cellular animals over the course of billions of years. That's a massive development. You could say that improvement is the purpose of evolution.

What evolution also tells us is that when animals adapt to their habitat their genes become 'tuned' to their surroundings. As the DNA tunes into signals like climate, terrain and available food, it comes to expect those signals from its surroundings and if these expectations are met then the animal expresses its full genetic potential for health.

This dance of the gene to the music of the environment takes many hundreds of generations to unfold, and the gene is constantly trying to keep rhythm, balance and harmony with the musical signals the environment creates. When the two are synchronised, it can be said that the animal has struck a sweet spot and because the genes are getting what they expect from their surroundings, the result is a state of growth and repair: a state of vitality.

Push the animal out of that sweet spot and you're now depriving the DNA of the environment and the signals it expects. Now stressors are being created and there is a mismatch between environment and DNA. In this contradiction the animal cannot grow and repair and is forced into defence and decay which leads to chronic disease.

We call signals that our genes expect 'biologically appropriate' and they are nutrients that feed our mind-body what it needs in order to thrive. These environmental signals trigger our genes to express growth and repair and when this happens we move toward vitality. But when we deprive our genes of these biologically appropriate signals, when we expose them to other, biologically inappropriate signals then we trigger our genes to express defence and decay. We've see this over and over again when animals are forced out of their ideal habitat or their habitat is damaged in some way: their health suffers.

In our universities, our homes and our minds we've separated ourselves from nature and elevated ourselves above it. We no longer pay attention to the basic laws of nature. We think that we can escape such laws and numb the warning signs as we continue to move away from nature's blueprint.

Ecosystem within an ecosystem
Our own health is forfeit to our arrogance, but so is that of our planet and the other life forms that coexist with us today. Damaging our own human ecosystem is reflected in the damage we wreak on the ecosystems we live in and depend on.

Our health is intimately linked with the health of the planet. Although the health of the biosphere we inhabit is outside the scope of this book I believe that only as we solve our internal incongruence will we really begin to solve the external ones. When we begin to save ourselves, we will begin to live in harmony with planet earth.

How does that shape our thinking?

It is curious to observe that animals in their natural habitat don't seem to develop chronic degenerative disease like heart disease, cancers, obesity, diabetes and ulcers. In the ground-breaking book *Why Zebras Don't Get Ulcers*, Dr Robert Sapolinsky explores why.

The basic premise of this research is that animals in their natural state have evolved over time to fit their environment and thrive. Their genes have changed through evolution to match the signals that their environment provides – their food, climate and surroundings. In this gene-environment match, we see health being expressed. This is the result of the dance the genes do to the music of the environment when they are in rhythm, balance and harmony.

In the wild, where genes and environment match, animals show very little to none of the chronic diseases that currently plague us so badly. Lions aren't depressed, giraffes don't develop diabetes, hippos, despite appearances, are not obese and elephants don't suffer chronic anxiety.

It's not completely understood but something curious happens in zoos. When we incarcerate wild animals in zoos we see some disturbing changes. Lions and tigers become listless and depressed; gorillas – despite the fact that they are vegetarians – develop high levels of cholesterol and heart disease. Animals in captivity develop diabetes, depression, infertility and low libido and have great difficulty breeding.

In the Cleveland Zoo in the USA, primate zookeepers noticed some problems with their gorillas, headed by a male called Mokolo. Mokolo, a Western Lowland gorilla native to Rwanda, had become overweight, developed high cholesterol and some signs of depression. Mokolo and his group had stopped grooming each other; in fact they were pulling their hair out, creating bald spots. They showed signs of anxiety, lost interest in sex and had dental problems. Most importantly, however, they were dying of heart disease. In fact, in the Cleveland Zoo and other US and foreign zoo's, heart disease was the leading cause of death amongst gorillas. But amongst wild gorillas heart disease was unheard of.

Mokolo wasn't smoking, he wasn't drinking, he wasn't eating fast food. He ate a 'balanced diet' based on the guidelines prescribed by the National Research Council that consisted of specially formulated gorilla biscuits.

The wild gorillas and Mokolo's gorilla troop are the same species and have exactly the same genes, so it couldn't be a genetic problem. The zookeepers looked at the gorillas in the wild and decided to try and recreate some of the natural conditions of wild gorillas within the zoo enclosure. Western Lowland gorillas in Rwanda eat green leafy plants all day and Mokolo's troop eats gorilla biscuits. The zookeepers decided to approximate the gorilla's natural diet.

They couldn't get exactly the same plants from Rwanda because it would have been too expensive so they visited their local supermarkets and collected vegetable and fruit leftovers for Mokolo's troop to try instead of gorilla biscuits. Within days they saw changes in the gorillas. They were cranky at first but then they started to get healthier and within weeks Mokolo's gorillas were transformed: their aggression died down; their anxiety and depression disappeared; they stopped pulling out their own hair; their grooming started again and they reconnected with each other; they moved around and played more and their fat melted.

Mokolo's blood tests confirmed that his cholesterol was coming down and his health was returning. What happened here is a really simple but powerful biological principle. The principle says that every animal has developed and evolved to thrive within a certain type of environment. Call it an environmental sweet-spot and that's made up of the physical, mental and chemical signals, just like our lifestyle is and it might be location and vegetation and temperature and light and predators and food and all of these different things. But now, when we take an animal away from its sweet spot, like putting it in a zoo and feeding it gorilla biscuits, we make their mind and their body force them to adapt, and shift into defence mode.

When we apply Mokolo's experience to ourselves we find heart disease and obesity and diabetes and cancer and depression and anxiety and learning problems and chronic pain and IBS and ADHD and many other issues. But if we feed an animal biologically appropriate foods as part of a vitalistic lifestyle, we can see health and vitality return. This concept has been replicated in zoos and enclosures worldwide and the results have been remarkable. This biological principle is true for all living things.

Why were the gorillas a bit cranky at first? The zookeepers later realised that this crankiness was nothing more than sugar withdrawal because the gorilla biscuits were so high in high fructose corn syrup!

The human zoo

I'm not suggesting we return to caves, live in loin cloths and let go of all the modern advances we've made since the dawn of civilisation. I like things such as my flushing toilet, my Apple MacBook and heating on a cold, stormy winter's night. I'm not saying that everything natural is good. Cyanide is a naturally occurring poison and I know that it can be fatal. I also don't pretend that life was perfect before we began our process of domestication around 10000 years ago. People who lived then, what I'll call wild free humans, died of things like trauma and infection – a broken leg could be fatal; things we don't consider deadly today if you are fortunate enough to live in the protection of industrialised society.

While our genes expect the sights, sounds, sensations, tastes and smells of our nature, our mind-body is bombarded by processed foods, pollution, the harsh noises of traffic and ringing phones, tar and tile underfoot, the stark look of symmetrical metals, bricks and mortar. Rarely are we in a situation where we see no sign of civilisation, hear no sound but perhaps that of leaves in a tree, feel nothing but earth between our toes or taste a complete meal devoid of additives, preservatives, flavourings or colourants.

This disconnect we've created shows itself in everything we do and in every aspect of our lives – our home and work, our children's school and our gym. 'Nature is meant to be outside' is what many of us have been conditioned to believe. Dirt is bad, fresh air is a luxury, vegetables must look a certain way, foods are best pre-packaged and pre-prepared and our movement is limited to periods of formal, isolated exercise on machines, if it's done at all.

Genetically we are almost identical to our caveman ancestors but in lifestyle there is absolutely no similarity. Genetic studies suggest that we have seen some modest genetic change in the last few thousand years. For example some groups of people developed enzymes to digest the sugar in milk as we domesticated cattle around 10 000 years ago. But this does not necessarily mean that they are completely adapted to dairy. Milk is a very complex set of chemicals and just because you can deal with one of them does not mean you're equipped to deal with the entire thing.

On an evolutionary scale, the changes we've made to our lifestyle have happened over a very short time. We've gone from being wild, free, hunter-gathering humans – which could be called our natural state – to domesticated humans in less than 10 000 years; the blink of an evolutionary eye. We've changed the music many times and our genes are off balance, out of rhythm and in a state of disharmony.

Like a caged lion pacing up and down behind bars, we shuttle back and forth from work and school in traffic knowing that there must be more. Like Mokolo's troop, we eat food that is a poor match for what our animal genes expect and we surrender our human potential and develop disease. Like any caged animal we've traded our freedom and vitality for a set of bars, only this time we did it to ourselves.

Where do animals thrive?

In *Why Zebras Don't Get Ulcers,* Dr Sapolinsky explores how a zebra on the savannah plains experiences stressors and contrasts it with how we as humans experience them.

A zebra in the grassy veld would experience stressors over a short period of time, usually lasting minutes or sometimes hours. Watching wildlife programmes I've seen many examples of how a lion, perfectly camouflaged in the long grass, stalks its black and white striped prey.

Cinematography in wildlife films is phenomenal as it can show in perfect detail the build up to the lion's attack, when and how the lion attacks, and whether the zebra is either caught and killed, or escapes and survives. Either way the incident of attack usually lasts minutes. This stressful event causes rapid changes in the physiology of the zebra to help it escape the clutches of the hungry lion. These changes are called the 'fight or flight' response and are the same changes you experience when you get a fright.

While I was writing this book I heard a loud crash of two cars colliding outside my house. Two cars had slammed into each other. A quick check on the occupants of both vehicles revealed no serious injuries but the Chiropractor in me observed that both sets of passengers were showing signs of the 'fight or flight' response. Both drivers were shaken and trembling; they had sweaty palms, pale faces and wide eyes; distracted attention; and had trouble recalling details of the crash.

This is what happens in both the zebra and you. The nervous system perceives some danger and prepares you to fight or run. The result is powerful:

- Your pupils dilate to allow more light in which improves your eyesight.
- Your body shifts blood and energy from the gut to your muscles – you don't need to digest food. This is also why you get a dry mouth when stressed because you don't need saliva to help digest food if you perceive that you are fighting for your life.
- Blood also moves from the frontal cortex, your rational, thinking part of your brain to your more primitive, instinctual brain, so reflexes, emotions and instinct take over from rational thought.
- Your heart beats faster and blood pressure goes up so you can move oxygen and energy around your body faster.
- Your blood sugar peaks to provide lots of short term energy.
- Your cholesterol goes up because it's the chemical foundation of your stress hormones and is very important in clotting and healing any wounds you might get in your fight to survive.
- Your immune system is depressed because it uses a lot of energy that is better spent getting away, and any infection can be fought later.
- Reproductive and growth hormones are shut down; there are energy-hungry systems that aren't needed when you're in survival mode.

This happens because of two changes in your body.

THE FIRST is the activation of a part of your nervous system that is responsible for the immediate fight or flight reaction. It's called the sympathetic nervous system. This fight or flight part of your nervous system sends messages directly to all your organs, telling them of danger, and tells the adrenal glands to release adrenalin immediately. Adrenalin in the blood stream is the short term chemical messenger of stress and signals the changes listed above. This first part happens in fractions of a second and does not last long.

THE SECOND happens when a part of your brain called the hypothalamus tells your pituitary gland to activate your adrenal glands. Here adrenalin is activated over a longer time and is released into the blood stream and continues to bathe every cell in your body with the message of acute stress. This pathway from your brain to your adrenals is called the HPA axis.

Between activation of your sympathetic (fight or flight) nervous system and your HPA axis you are now ready to face your threat. In the case of both the zebra and humans, in our animal state, all of these changes are intelligent in the short term and they give us the best chance of surviving a potentially deadly situation. This is our defence mode at work, helping us to survive and get away from the stressful environment.

If after a few minutes we are still experiencing stress then a new phase of adaptation kicks in when the brain tells the adrenals to release cortisol – a powerful hormone. It takes over from adrenalin and can result in further adaptation over a longer period of time. If this phase persists because of chronic exposure to stressors then we begin to get the chemicals of stress that wreak havoc on your mind-body. The result is chronic inflammation.

If, however it's a short term threat then once the stress is survived and the stress response passes, the zebra's physiology returns to normal and so does yours.

In the case of the accident outside our house, my wife and I sat with one of the drivers while she called her husband and processed the event; within a few minutes her trembling stopped and she became calmer and the colour returned to her face. The lingering effects of the shock would last for a while longer but the worst was over.

This stress pathway that helps in life or death situations is also triggered in social situations: your looming deadline, your best client telling you that they are cancelling their account, knowing that you won't be able to pay your home loan this month, suspecting that your spouse is being unfaithful, having your mother in law come to stay or even having a big test at school.

Physical injury can set off the stress response too: first responders to a car accident often have to manage both the injury and check if the person is going into shock. This state of 'shock' is the stress response magnified.

You can also set off this pathway when you have a much lower grade of stress. Simply spending hours sitting down can propagate a stress response, not in the same way as a car accident, but in much more insidious almost invisible way.

96

Almost as invisible, the pollution in your air, water and food can create a low grade response from your mind-body. The things we choose to eat and drink can do the same. Over time these low grade stressors accumulate and can create a slow motion disaster for your well-being and your life's potential.

Through the course of evolution zebras have evolved to suit their habitat so their genes and their environment match. Their DNA is programmed to respond to the stimuli that the savannah brings and to produce homeostasis, health and well-being as a result. Their innate programming expects short term stressors that they can then recover from; it makes them stronger.

Their balance in nature isn't a static one. Through the seasons there is fluctuation in the availability of food, in the numbers of zebra in the herds, in how much fat each zebra stores and many other factors. These variations are also expected by their DNA.

If you observe zebra over the course of a few years you'd notice that the herd is dependent on so many factors in their ecosystem, from the weather to the availability of good grazing ground, from the number of lions hunting them to the quality of soil they live on and a whole host more. They are in a dynamic balance with their environment and their health depends on that delicate equilibrium.

From this perspective we see a finely balanced dance happening. The homeostasis inside the zebra that leads to a state of thriving is dependent on the external balance of the environment, which in turn depends on the internal balance of each other living part of the ecosystem. When the animal is in harmony with its surroundings in the dynamic dance we can say that it exists in its evolutionary sweet spot. The further from that sweet spot it's forced to be, the more it has to adapt and the more it has to adapt the more it experiences ill health.

There are so many moving parts in the equation of the zebra's well-being that we would be mistaken to focus on just a few of them. Speak to the best ecologists in the world and they will tell you that we understand precious little about the intertwined interactions that happen in nature. What these experts will tell you, though, is that the best we can do when managing natural ecosystems is to mimic nature whenever possible.

This is the lesson we learned from Alan Savory when he realised that only by following nature's blueprint could he help to heal and regenerate grasslands. The same is true of the ecosystem and animal in you and I, too.

When do animals become chronically sick?

The word homeostasis means 'standing at the same level' which implies that a system is static or uniform all the time but, in reality, life is always in flux. In recent time scientists have moved toward a more dynamic way of thinking about how our mind-body stays in balance.

Dr Bruce McKewan of the Rockefeller University is one of the world's leading experts on how the body adapts under stressful conditions to maintain its internal balance. He coined the term allostasis, which translates to 'remaining stable by being variable.'

Allostasis then is the study of persistent stress and how it affects your mind-body. It tells us that we have a certain 'adaptive potential' that Dr McEwen has called the General Adaptive Potential or GAP. Just like an elastic band can stretch so far before it snaps, so your physiology can adapt to a certain amount of 'allostatic load' before defence gives way to decay.

In *The Wellness and Prevention Paradigm*, Dr James Chestnut likens the allostatic load to small stones in our backpack. Each one we accumulate makes our load heavier, pulling our health down, pushing us further into adaptation and bringing us closer to disease and decay. Each rock activates more of our stress pathways and taxes our mind-body.

Our response to accumulated stress, or 'allostasis', goes through three phases: first comes alarm where we have our fight or flight reaction. If this persists we have the second phase: adaptation. Here our mind-body systems begin to trade short term comfort for long term survival. We can see how this might work in our iceberg analogy where developing frostbite to preserve our body temperature helps us survive longer and give us a better chance at survival.

Unlike the zebra on the savannah plains that can escape the mental and emotional stress of the lion by running away, zoo animals are confined 24/7. They experience the same cascade of biological responses the wild zebra does but they suffer them over a longer period of time. Their smart, short term responses that were innately programmed into their DNA over millions of years do not have the ability to meet this new problem.

As we layer on more stressors and accumulate more allostatic load throughout our lives we do exactly the same thing to ourselves. We live in human zoos of our own creation that are fraught with stressors.

Short term defensive solutions that once allowed survival, and even made the animal stronger, now cause decay, degeneration and lead to disease. Here's how this would play out for you:

1. Shifting blood away from the gut causes problems with digestion and absorption of foods. Many chronic diseases have some of their roots in gut health.
2. Allowing your primitive, instinctual brain to take the reins makes you more reactive, irrational and emotional – anxiety or depression dominate and libido wanes. It shortens your attention and concentration span, affects your moods and your ability to form and hold memories.
3. Chronically high blood pressure damages your heart and arteries and can lead to heart disease and strokes.
4. Constant spikes and troughs in your blood sugar and hormones causes damage to your heart, brain, arteries, reproductive system and much more.
5. The damage to your heart and arteries with the accumulation of cholesterol to try and repair it can lead to blood clots causing strokes and heart attacks.
6. Chronic stressors damage the immune system. It releases the chemicals of chronic stress and chronic inflammation is the result.

> Chronic inflammation shrinks your brain, shreds your arteries, cannibalises your muscles, demineralises your bones, imbalances your hormones, distress your gut and inflames your immune system.

This chronic build up, or allostatic load, happens in nature and it presents us with a cautionary tale. Every year salmon swim upstream through the rivers to spawn or reproduce. They battle the currents, rocks and predators for many miles to make their way back to their breeding ground. These brave creatures do this to ensure that they fertilise a new generation of salmon – and then they die.

The fish are killed by their own stress response. While it gives them tremendous surges of energy needed for the upward journey, in the end it builds up to toxic levels. Short term stress response (defence) can be very useful but chronic stress response (decay) causes damage and death.

Our chronic stress

Our food is more and more artificial; laced with chemicals only recently invented with unknown long-term effects on our health. Where we once ate off the land and had foods that were local and seasonal and unprocessed, we now have pre-packaged and artificial foods, covered with fertilisers, herbicides and pesticides. Many of these 'foods' we now consume didn't even exist a few decades ago, never mind the 10 000 years it's been since we began farming.

Human animals enjoyed a variety of activity from lifting and dragging heavy things to jumping and climbing, from sprinting to hanging out in a squat position for hours. Since the industrial revolution our long hours in the sitting position has been cited as the 'new smoking' for our generation and is associated with obesity, diabetes, depression, chronic pain and cancer. Our movement has become stifled, regimented and constricted in the form of occasional exercise. Our bodies have become structurally distorted, affecting posture and putting increased stress on our nervous systems.

To borrow from Bilbo Baggins in *The Lord of the Rings*, mentally and emotionally we're like, "Too little butter spread over too much toast." It's been estimated that today, we experience in the space of a single day the mental stress a person 200 years ago was exposed to over two years. We are bombarded with information from our computers, our smart phones, our tablets, our radios, our TVs, and everyone is clamouring for our attention.

Amongst many of my professional friends, their email inbox is a significant source of anxiety. This didn't even exist until the 1990's. Back then we would have been intimately associated with a smaller number of people whom we phoned or wrote to. We are now Facebook friends with hundreds, but close to none. When we would once have had the time to enjoy a considerable amount of down-time we now live in an era of immediate gratification – 'I want it now' – and are pulled in every direction by all the urgent priorities we accept.

> *Every stress leaves and indelible scar,*
> *and the organism pays for its survival after a stressful situation*
> *by becoming a little older.*
> PROF HANS SELYE PhD

Each of these daily stressors drives our system further and further into adaptation and defence, eventually pushing us into a state of fatigue where we get closer to decay and disease. Each of us has a different stress load and each of us will respond in our own way to each stressor, so we will not all suffer the same consequences from the same stressors.

What about bigger more acute stressors like physical injury, loss of loved ones or acutely poisonous foods and infections? If smaller stressors are like small stones, these big stressors are more akin to rocks or boulders in your backpack. Acute stressors like these are bound to affect you and bring you down. How well you absorb them and how quickly you recover is largely determined by how full your backpack was when they came along.

Modern medicine is beginning to realise this now and we see it when, instead of only focusing on *re*habilitation after a surgery, enlightened doctors are now working on *pre*habilitation before the event to improve outcomes afterwards. That's the same as working on unloading the backpack so that the added load of the surgery affects the person less and improves their recovery afterwards.

How do you help chronically sick animals become well

Take nature's lead
Applying the lens of evolution to your health is a useful way of improving your well-being and quality of life. By addressing all dimensions of stress – how we eat, move, think, rest, get exposed to nature and breathe – and adding in the nutrients that human animals would have been exposed to has given rise to a whole field of research called evolutionary or ancestral health care.

Applying the evolutionary model to health care has caused quite a stir in mainstream medicine as it tends to undermine the conventional approach. Using this approach, chronic, degenerative diseases are being reversed, incurable lifestyle diseases are resolved and medications that were supposed to be for life are ditched as people rediscover the innate intelligence within us.

Wild, free human animals existed before the agricultural revolution about 10 000 years ago. Before that we lived as hunter-gatherers and lived an interesting life. Without sanitation and emergency medical care their existence could be seen as backwards, but there are a few surprising things that come out of their histories.

It would probably surprise you to know that we were healthy living in our natural habitat, surrounded by the signals our genes had evolved over millions of years.

Evidence has shown that chronic and degenerative conditions hardly existed, even among our elderly. We had a varied and incredibly nutrient-rich diet of locally sourced food which was biologically appropriate. We enjoyed active lifestyles with varied movements and our physical conditioning would rival that of Olympic decathletes today.

From our contact with modern groups of people relatively untouched by modern civilisation we know that their levels of happiness are high with little mental stress, especially the type that lasts days, months and years, like ours. We were connected, cohesive, egalitarian societies that are a far cry from the disconnection, segregation and estrangement we see in society today.

When we hear that wild, free humans led lives that were 'poor, nasty, brutish and short', we're hearing the voices of the mechanists who separate mind and body and declared humans as above nature. The mechanists reject the natural in favour of dominion over the natural world.

We're also told that the average life expectancy of Palaeolithic humans was approximately 35 years old and that none lived much longer than that. While it is true that the *average* life expectancy might have been about 35, this number needs to be put into perspective: if a child dies at birth or in the first few years of life then the age of this child distorts the average downward. Estimates vary but on the low end approximately 20% of people in these societies lived well into their 60's and were active, productive members of their society.

The Agricultural Revolution (350 generations ago)
As we started farming our stature dropped by as much as 5 inches in height. Skeletal records show that we developed thinner bones, arthritis and more dental problems, but most notably we lived *shorter* lives at an average of 20 years. Our diet suffered as nutrient rich animals and plants were replaced increasingly by nutrient

poor grains. Not only were we decaying as we lived and dying sooner, but also developed a whole new set of health problems. Mummified remains in Egypt, close to the heart of the agricultural revolution in the Middle East, show signs of diseases like cancer and gout. These conditions had hardly existed before we domesticated plants like wheat and began farming them.

Instead of having hours of downtime, living in an egalitarian society of up to 150 members and enjoying life as our hunter-gatherer ancestors did, we worked the land for days on end and suffered crippling health conditions. We began congregating in towns and cities and our communal waste and poor hygiene caused even more health problems. Infectious diseases could run rampant, wiping out entire cities at a time.

It wasn't all bad though. Across the world culture developed in tandem with our civilisation even as chronic and degenerative conditions became more common. Dental health is very closely related to degenerative diseases and general health. Dental records show that following the development of agriculture and building of cities, our dental health declined considerably.

The Industrial Revolution (7 generations ago)
The next big change for our species was the industrial revolution. Originating in the British Empire and spreading around the globe we began harnessing machine power to do the tasks of men and women. Fewer people doing manual labour meant more people sitting and working behind desks. Once again our lives were transformed and taken still further away from the stimuli our genes expected. We were less mobile and had ready access to refined foods that we produced in bulk with mechanisation.

Wheat flour became our staple diet in Europe and sugar became more and more common. As the European empires spread so did their farming and food processing. Health and dental records show another decline in our health, reports of conditions like cancer increased, and diabetes became a more common condition. Just before the start of the Industrial Revolution life expectancy in London was 18.

We inflicted our 'civilisation' on traditional cultures around the world. White men with white flour and white sugar, white doctors in white coats with white pills wreaked havoc on the health of the 'natives.' The 'whitey blight' did more harm than good in many colonies. In two generations the Inuit from Northern America, who in their traditional lifestyle had very rare cases of obesity and cancers, developed rates of these diseases proportionate to those of westerners as they adopted our lifestyles. Early records show that when Native Americans were hunter gatherers only about one in a hundred of them had diabetes. In 2011 it was one in two.

Sanitation, more than any other innovation, has improved our health and longevity allowing us to live in towns and cities and our life expectancy to rise up to about 75 years. Before sewers and flushing toilets were common, infectious diseases could ravage whole towns, cities and regions. In the Dark Ages a lack of hygiene allowed the Black Plague to spread throughout Europe, killing nearly 30% of the population of Europe. The Spanish Flu of 1918 spread from the gangrenous trenches of the First World War and killed up to 5% of the world's population.

The advent of antibiotics allowed us to fight some infections and anaesthetics allowed us to perform better surgeries and these two things have saved many lives and have helped to improved our life expectancy.

It's important to note that, apart from developed nations, in much of the world access to basic sanitation and emergency medical care is sorely lacking and many people are subjected to poor standards of living and severe health problems.

The Chemical Revolution (3 generations ago)
The next revolution to shape our civilisation and move us further from the signals our genes expect was the Chemical Revolution following the Second World War. The machines of war began to produce plastics, fertilisers and all sorts of other useful chemicals. Over the last 70 years we've unleashed these chemicals on our world without much thought to either our health or that of the planet.

Estimates vary but about 150 000 new chemicals have been created. Many of these have never been tested for their long term effects on our health and that of other animals, plants and ecosystems. In our arrogance we once again believed we could conquer nature with our new technology.

Some of the chemicals we have produced promised to control swarms of insects that ate our crops and spread disease and we sprayed with reckless abandon. DDT was one of these chemicals and it did kill insects but unfortunately it also wrecked ecosystems when it caused birds to lay eggs with thin shells and decimated huge populations of birds, including the condor and the bald eagle. DDT is now a recognised carcinogen which disrupts the hormonal system in humans, too. This is just one example of thousands of chemicals that have been deemed safe, only to later have been proven dangerous.

Each new chemical in our food, water and air might not be that much of a worry on its own because we may be capable of dealing with small doses of them with little cost to our health. Starting in the mother's womb it's the accumulation of these toxins over the course of our lives and generations that can cause real damage.

In a study of the placenta, directly after childbirth, over 287 different but known toxic chemicals were detected. These are toxins that have made their way into the pregnant mother's body to the unborn child. The developing foetus is particularly sensitive to the chemical signals it receives from its mother. Minute changes can lead to tragic deformities.

More subtle are the cumulative effects of the swathes of synthesised compounds that we add to the stew after conception. Our ancient biology does not have the tools to fight this kind of stress and so the ultimate outcome is more defence and more decay at a younger age.

New chemicals pervade your life and while some are avoidable, some are not. They preserve, flavour, colour and 'enhance' your food and the places your food is grown. Your cosmetics are full of them and you readily absorb a lot of what you put on your skin. Researchers call this the 'body burden' of chemicals.

One study analysed the urine and blood of 20 teenage girls and found that they each had between 10 and 15 chemicals from their cosmetic products in their body. These chemicals are known to disrupt the hormonal system. The researchers could only test for 25 chemicals while, on average, each girl was exposed to 174 unique chemicals in 17 personal care products.

The tap water we drink is infused with hormones and antibiotics and our air is visibly polluted. Drugs, both prescribed and pushed are administered from birth with little attention paid to their cumulative effects through life. Your home and office are bathed in compounds from paint to fire retardants that have probably been linked to diseases.

The most remote parts of the Pacific Ocean are contaminated by fire retardants, fertilisers and plastics so our chemical concoctions are everywhere. We are infused with these from the very start of our lives and we don't know what the long term effects of chronic, low dose, cumulative chemicals are.

Another study looked at four mothers and their four daughters and found that each person's blood and urine was contaminated by 35 chemicals on average. The chemicals were from furniture, cosmetics, fabrics and other consumer products and had never been tested for safety.

Like unsupervised children with new toys humanity has created a cornucopia of new compounds and then let them steep into our mind-body without knowing the consequences. While many of these chemicals have some benefit there still remain more questions than answers about the safety of these chemicals.

The Information Revolution (2 generations ago)
The most recent revolution which most of us have experienced is the Information Revolution. More than anything else, the rise of the desk bound job has sedated and robbed us of the vital stimulation that movement creates. A survey by the Chiropractic Association of Australia indicated that the amount of time that the average Australian is not sitting down to work, commute, eat and watch TV is 73 minutes. The Aussies are generally known for being active but this is only an hour and 13 minutes a day spent actually moving in any way!

Sitting is now being called the smoking of this generation because of its link to poor health. If you accumulate 4 or more hours of sitting a day then your risk of conditions like cancer, heart disease, diabetes, chronic pain and depression sky rocket. The bad news is that the exercise we do in the gym a few hours a week doesn't necessarily undo the damage created by sitting!

With the increase in information there has been a decrease in our ability to handle it. The stream of information that we're exposed to from the TV, radio, email, surfing the web, social media, the news, and billboards is phenomenal.

We seem to be more time-poor than ever before and even struggle to find time to do any kind of activity, which is usually artificial and limited exercise in a gym. We don't seem to have the time to source, prepare, cook and eat real food. Instead we rely on pre-packaged food substitutes; the poor cousins of what our genes expect.

While we have hundreds of friends on Facebook we feel more and more isolated as individuals and less and less connected to the people around us. On a trip to London I was astonished to notice how, even though people were physically close, they were mentally and emotionally withdrawn. On the underground tube system almost everyone has headphones on and move like pre-programmed automatons. The person who makes eye contact or smiles, which is usually me, is frowned upon.

In suburbia the situation is no better. How many of us know and have good relations with our neighbours? They're usually the strangers next door that do odd things that annoy us.

Our relationships suffer as we chase low value material goals. Our human values suffer as we get caught up in yet another drama involving heroes and villains of our own making. We worry about politics and things far out of our control when our families and friends are right in front of us, being neglected.

Biologically, we are still hunter-gatherers expecting the cues of the savannah for how we eat, move and think. Our genes expect these cues and are primed to create a state of growth and repair when they sense a growth environment. Instead we're like the gorilla in the zoo: completely out of place and degenerating rapidly.

It's not all bad news. While it's important to realise that we are not in good shape and that the consequences of staying the same are dire, like Mokolo the gorilla, nature has allowed for our revival and left clues telling us what to do. By studying success and following the trail of breadcrumbs it leaves behind we can reclaim our lives, rekindle our passion and experience freedom, connection and live bigger lives.

Remember that our genes are primed to respond to environmental signals from our evolutionary sweet spot and, in response, they activate growth and repair our mind-body. If we can find out what is biologically appropriate for humans and then use that as a guideline for a vitalistic lifestyle then we have a chance of re-activating our wellness genes. ●

Nature cannot be commanded except by being obeyed.
SIR FRANCIS BACON

6

Vitality is inside-out

You can't be the solution.
Antioxidants can hurt you.
3 Paths – Which are you on?
Falling into fat-loss.
Your allostatic fingerprint.

How do we currently view health care?

By now you get the idea that many of our fundamental beliefs around our health and well-being are not serving us and are potentially hurting us. We have also visited the truths about health; where it comes from and how it works.

Allopathic Beliefs	Vitalistic Beliefs
Not sick = healthy	Health = optimum function
You are a machine	You are an ecosystem
You are broken	You are innately intelligent
You are separate from nature	You are an animal

How does that shape our thinking?

The myths we've allowed ourselves to believe tend to make us passive in our approach to our well-being. We wait to get sick or to experience some problem before we take action to improve our health. We sacrifice our potential to live full, active and vibrant lives and instead live lives of quiet desperation.

The idea that we can best understand ourselves by separating ourselves into ever smaller parts is well entrenched in our psyche. When you use this approach your mind is separate from your body and your body is simply a mechanistic collection of organic goo that ticks. If parts wear out or break you can easily fix them or slot in new ones. The real issue is that we don't measure the consequences of our actions in terms of the price our mind-body has to pay because we think that it can be fixed later, with a pill or surgery.

Such a flawed belief makes it easy to play the role of the victim. Since we believe that things beyond our control determine our level of health, we can't blame ourselves for our state of well-being. That's a comforting thought but it has a counterpoint – we can't be the solution either. In this level of thinking we need someone or something outside of us to rescue us.

In the face of health care challenges we adopt the victim mentality which reinforces the passive approach that got us into the situation in the first place and now we're chasing our tails. The never ending cycle of victimhood enslaves us all – slaves to the next quick fix, the next guru promising salvation, the priesthood of white coats ordained to solve our ills. The problem is not outside; it is not well-intentioned people and professionals. The problem lies inside.

The myths are comforting, though, like a bedtime story where the good guys always win. Being the master of nature exalts us above her, making us no longer subject to her rules. Since we've trumped natural forces we no longer need to pay attention to our place in the landscape. Enticed by our own ingenuity we've rebelled against our biology, hoping to escape the consequences like a teenager missing their curfew and thinking their parents can't hear them climbing in the window at 2 am. As for the teenager, there are always consequences. For us they are cumulative and so can be practically invisible for a time. As we accumulate these invisible layers of stressors to which our body must adapt through defence physiology, we erode our human potential.

What is the result?
Taking the passive approach invariably means that we wait too long to take action and suffer some irreparable damage as a result. When we do act, we tend to take the shortcut and address only the symptom and not its cause. If we had a leaking roof we'd probably use a bucket to contain the water, but when the rain stops and the roof is no longer leaking, have we fixed the problem? The roof will leak again when it next rains, other leaks may develop and the damp will seep unseen through the structure of the house, rotting it away from the inside. We have simply perpetuated the problem.

Since we view ourselves as machines with parts that can be fixed or replaced we tend to focus on immediate performance and ignore longevity. We consume our internal health resources as problems arise, but with no regard to the cumulative effect these problems may lead to. We think we have magical technicians who can work on us and fix everything with drugs or surgery and if our technicians can't solve the problem then it's unsolvable.

In life, we are either empowered or disempowered. If we choose to play the role of the disempowered victim we will attract overpowering persecutors to fill that role. What is a victim without a persecutor? When a victim is being taken advantage of they need a rescuer like a knight in shining armour on his white steed to make all the ills of the world go away. The problem can be that the rescuer becomes another persecutor to justify the victim's need for turmoil. How many times have we praised doctors for helping us, only to curse them later for the unintended consequences of our earlier salvation?

A not uncommon question we hear when we go through the results of our initial set of tests is, "Why did none of the other doctors tell me this was going to happen!?" The answer is that either they didn't even know or, if they did, they didn't know what else to do. They are stuck in a system that has no answers to the problems it has created.

If we're waiting to be rescued then we're waiting in vain. Some of those that we hope will be our saviours are motivated by profit and not your well-being. Even true health care providers with the best intentions will help, coach and encourage you, but they're not going to save you. Only you can save yourself.

How is vitality different?

The new model of Thrive! provides a map to help you navigate your way from the barren desert of ill-being toward the oasis of well-being. With Thrive! instead of treating illness, you reactivate your wellness genes and create health.

Knowing that merely existing or surviving is not your default state is exciting. Vitality is a higher state of being that you both deserve and can attain: more energy, greater focus, increased ease, a better physical condition and higher levels of personal performance.

Realising that you are the hero of your own story and that the potential for your well-being is within you like a seed waiting to germinate is incredibly empowering.

You can Thrive! by switching on your wellness genes. It will not happen any other way. All your genes need are the right nutrients in what you eat, how you move and think. There's no quick fix bucket under the leak; you will have to allow your genes time to reactivate your mind-body and your health to blossom.

The belief that you are an integrated being, more than the sum of your parts, gives you an empowering and inspiring, totally new perspective on your life. Knowing this raises your level of thought, inspires great actions and infuses courage and a strong will.

Seeing the order in nature, from the quantum to the cosmic and the organic in between, and your place in it, shines a peaceful light on your being. It gives you space to breathe. Recognising that you are whole and part of a greater whole allows you to be proactive about your well-being. Honouring the natural blueprint within you gives you a framework to begin working with, instead of fumbling in the dark. It is the foundation of your vitality.

It's inside-out

Antioxidants are chemicals that your mind-body uses for defence and clean up. They combat a process called oxidative stress by removing volatile molecules called free radicals that, if left to accumulate unchecked, age the body and can damage cell structure and DNA, or kill cells. Oxidative stress is the process that weakens living things and allows them to succumb to disease, makes them age and decay – it is associated with over 100 different diseases including cancer and heart disease. Antioxidants seemed to be able to protect us from a whole host of diseases and be 'anti-ageing'.

With this thought in mind we began to supplement our diets with antioxidants like Vitamin E and beta carotene. We thought that if some was good then more must be better. Since these antioxidants came from external sources and weren't made in our body we call them *exogenous*. Unfortunately, with time and research, it was found that these synthetic exogenous antioxidants weren't helpful and could even be harmful. Some were even found to increase the risk of death in those who took them. It seemed as though there was a lot more to the whole picture. The complexity of the ecosystem and the limitation of the mechanistic mindset had reared its head again.

What is much more powerful, though, is activating your body's own ability to create *endogenous* antioxidants. Endogenous antioxidants are more powerful and your mind-body intelligently produces them in the right quantity at the right time depending on what type of free radicals are present.

Once again we see that health is not about trying to micromanage the function of your 75 trillion cell ecosystem. It's about addressing any interference to your body's ability to manage itself and then standing back and letting it do what it needs to do.

The principles

There are three basic scenarios of where you may be right now, and although the principles for transformation are the same for each scenario, the way you apply them might be different.

1. **You are below the line**, experiencing symptoms and need to make changes fast. Here you live a paradox: change is hard but drastic change is necessary. Your mind-body has been hijacked by supernormal stimuli (see The Weakness in Your Genes) that have short circuited your evolutionary programming, creating addiction-like behaviour that is hard to break. In this scenario 'cold turkey' can be extremely effective: you are motivated by the pain and suffering of your symptoms which is a powerful driving force, but staying power is critical. Once you move up to Scenario 2, however, you won't be suffering as much anymore. New drivers that give you inspiration to maintain lifestyle change can help you avoid relapse and follow your inspiration: This is your 'Guiding Why'.

2. **You are above the line** but you are far from being well. You might carry a little more fat on your thighs or around the middle, your movement isn't free and your headspace is not especially clear. Here you have the opportunity to make sure you don't create any long term damage. But without the pain and suffering of symptoms to drive you, you need to find what you're missing in life, your source of inspiration, your 'Guiding Why'. The fear of getting worse and relapsing is also a strong driver and can be harnessed to keep you moving up toward vitality.

3. **There is no line**. Here you are inspired by the fullness of your experience of life, your energy, drive and focus. Your body feels great and you feel like you look good naked. You probably won't look like a model from a magazine, but more like a wild, free human. You move freely and have confidence in your mind-body to handle what life throws at you. Here your drive comes from your inspiration to be more connected; your belief that you could be refining and optimising your experience of life. Your fear of losing this state of vitality can also be a strong motivator, so use that feeling to keep you on your toes.

Take control of the choices you make every day by eating, moving and thinking in ways that nurture your innate resistance and decrease your stress load. **Start now.**

How does vitality work?

Sprouting health

When I was about 12 we did an experiment in school. It involved putting a broad bean in some moist cotton wool and watching and documenting the process of germination and growth into a plant.

We all compared notes about who saw their first shoot and when this happened and whose was growing faster. My broad bean seed didn't seem to want to germinate and I thought that either I had done something wrong or the seed was a dud.

Some of my classmates were in the same predicament and tried different things to get their beans to grow. Some used fertiliser, or special sun lamps and others were dong crazy things like adding odd chemicals that their parents used to fertilise plants and kill bugs in their garden!

My teacher took me aside when she saw how despondent I was. She was a real gem of a teacher, smart, funny and pretty, too, and all the boys had a crush on her. She told me how, when she was my age, her seed had been late in sprouting, too. What she did was to take extra special care of it. She made sure it had just enough water but not too much, enough cotton wool but not too much, enough light but not too much. She paid extra attention to the seed and even talked to it. She gave it everything it needed and then gave it something else, something very special. She gave it time. When everyone else was boasting about how many leaves their bean plant had, she just went home and took care of her little seed with patience and with the certainty that this little thing would grow.

Eventually my teacher's seed did sprout and it grew beautifully, in fact she had replanted it in her mother's garden and said that it was still there to this day. She said, "Greg, you have to *allow* the seed to sprout, you can't *force* it." Well, with that pep talk I was dedicated to my little seed. I made extra sure it had just enough water, adequate sunlight and the right amount of cotton wool – and then I gave it time, I waited. I knew that inside this little bean was a whole green plant ready to explode and that I had to be patient.

Sure enough my seed did sprout and in just a few days I had a plant with a few big, broad leaves that I could boast about too. What we realised in this experiment is that you can't force a seed to germinate. Some seeds grow fast and some grow slow but as long as the seed was undamaged, it *would* grow. All the seed needed was the right ingredients and time.

The road to vitality and Thrive! is much like *allowing* that bean to grow. You need all the right ingredients: an integrated brain and body and vitalistic nutrition, movement and headspace. You also need time. You need patience. Some beans will grow faster than others and some people will get results faster than others, too.

Know that your spark of life is not beyond repair, you are not a damaged bean. Inside of you is a spark of life that can help you grow, repair and heal. The damage you may have done in the past might limit how much healing you can do, but it is never too late and you are never too sick to start now.

CASE HISTORY 5:
Falling Asleep

JEFF IS THE CEO of a large company. He came to me for coaching because he wanted to take his personal performance to the next level. Jeff's main problem was not being able to sleep properly. He would lie awake at night and try his best to fall asleep. He would try so hard that it frustrated him to the point that he would get up and go and watch TV or work on his computer. From the outside Jeff seemed to be in reasonable condition: he was in the gym a few times a week, he wasn't obese and he put on a good mask so people thought he was quite happy.

To a trained eye, however, a few things stood out. His skin was blotchy, he had digestive bloating, his libido was low and, despite the gym routine, his strength was waning and his waistline was slowly expanding.

Jeff wanted to start with techniques to get him to fall asleep. After doing a full assessment of his lifestyle it became clear that, while falling asleep was Jeff's primary symptom, the cause lay elsewhere. His internal rhythm and cycles were out of sync and this can affect sleep patterns, resulting in either sleeplessness or fitful, interrupted sleep. To remedy this we had to *allow* his mind-body to sleep again, but we couldn't *force* it. Jeff was used to getting his own way and he wanted to find something that would force him to sleep.

He'd tried sleeping pills and, although they rendered him unconscious, he didn't feel rested in the mornings and sometimes felt even worse than if he had just tossed and turned the whole night. I mentioned that hypnotic techniques might help him to quiet his brain, but this would just mask the underlying problem. We made a deal that we would try addressing the underlying issue for 2 weeks and then use the hypnotic techniques if necessary.

Jeff followed my advice during week 1: he made some changes to his eating, moving and thinking habits and began to get his spine and nervous system checked by a Chiropractor. He began to feel a change: he slept better most nights and felt more rested most mornings.

By week 2 Jeff was feeling noticeably better and happy with the process. His internal rhythm was so deranged that he had to work with this new routine for some months before he felt he was back in control. Without using hypnosis, a year or so later Jeff told me that things were great and getting progressively better still. He realised that he had a lot of healing to do and that he was a completely different man.

Moving toward vitality is a lot like falling asleep. You have to have the right conditions – called sleep hygiene – a nice quiet space, a comfortable bed and pillow and a dark room at a slightly lower temperature. You also need to allow your mind-body to wind up during the day – the awakened cycle – and then wind down to begin entering the sleeping cycle.

Doing some movement and being outside in the sun early during the day lifts you up, and then primes you to wind down later on as the light fades. Eating foods and timing meals that work with your innate daily rhythms and cycles helps you stay awake and alert for the day and then rest and recuperate at night. Having a habit of mental and emotional awareness lets you know when to press on and work hard, when you need to take a step back and rest during the day, and when a few days or weeks of rest might be needed.

All of this preparation is already built-in when you eat, move and think in biologically appropriate or vitalistic ways, but you can't make good sleep happen without the right sleep hygiene. You still have to *fall* asleep. You can prepare during the day and you can arrange at night but it's is still a process of allowing sleep to happen rather than *making* it happen. Your mind-body knows how to fall asleep and it will never forget. Problems arise, however, when there is an imbalance in our lifestyle which inhibits the sleep *process*.

Falling into vitality

Your mind-body knows how to access growth and repair; it knows the journey of vitality to the state of Thrive! All we have to do is balance the system, remove blockages and then allow health to return. Like germinating a seed or like falling asleep some people need less attention than others. Some of us have seeds of health that need a little more time and a little more attention. Like seeds and like sleep we cannot force ourselves into vitality. It is a process.

What your mind-body needs to be able to germinate its innate seeds of health are purity and sufficiency of your biologically required nutrients in your lifestyle and clear function of your nervous system. What imbalances the system and blocks your full expression of health and light is deficiency and toxicity in the way you eat, move and think, and dysfunction of your nervous system.

Addressing dysfunction, toxicities and deficiencies will allow your mind-body to begin the process of growth and repair. You may need to allow yourself time to regenerate; in a forest that has been logged you can't just plant the trees and expect the forest to flourish straight way. You have to replant the trees, encourage the animals to come back and then allow the process of re-integration and regeneration to happen.

Falling into weight loss

Weight loss or weight management is everyone's hot topic and one that comes up with my clients every day. In my seminars I often ask, "What's the fastest way to lose 20kgs?" Usual answers are: this diet or that diet. Sometimes someone mentions fasting or even acquiring a tummy bug that causes vomiting and diarrhoea; you'd be surprised at how many times this suggestion comes up!

Some of these 'solutions' might work, but they are not the fastest. The fastest way to lose 20kg is to amputate a body part! For an adult, their thigh, leg and foot make up just under 20% of their body weight. So if you weigh 100kg, after an amputation you will weigh 80kg. Does this make you healthier or slimmer?

Weight loss, or more accurately 'fat loss', is subject to the same principle of *allowing* rather than *forcing*. It is something your mind-body knows how to do and hasn't just forgotten. Imbalances in your ecosystem are causing defence physiology that result in fat accumulation and can make it a challenge to shift the excess fat.

You can temporarily starve yourself into weight loss but if you haven't allowed your mind-body to move into growth and repair, if you haven't begun the journey to vitality, then you might be fooling the scale for a while but you're not going to improve your life.

Each of us has a unique allostatic load

Each person has a unique allostatic load affecting their mind-body, and how much of this load each of us can adapt to is different. Professor McEwen calls this our General Adaptive Potential (GAP). Within that, each part of our ecosystem has different amounts of stress that they can adapt to – there is variance between people and there is variance within people too! This is why people respond in different ways to different stressors and because of this we are individually different.

This is the reason why one person can smoke their entire life and live to 90 while another might die of lung cancer at 50. In this example it's wise to realise that the person who lived to 90 may have suffered other consequences of their habit and probably did not unlock their full human potential, which would have enabled them to live a fuller, happier and richer life had they not smoked. Just because they didn't develop a disease does not mean they were healthy.

The differences in health and appearance in genetically identical twins comes down to epigenetics: the way your mind-body turn genes on and off. Dr Bruce Lipton who did experiments with the stem cells in the petri dishes and cells with identical DNA would do different things depending on which dish they were placed in. It was the environment, not the genes that mattered most.

I've know athletes who could party 5 nights a week drinking, smoking and doing drugs into the early hours of the morning, and then still turn up to practices and matches and turn in stellar performances. People like me, on the other hand, had to work hard just to make the 'C' team. Our ecosystems adapted to our lifestyle stressors in different ways. We can't assume that those partying athletes were healthy and they usually suffered frequent injuries and had much shorter careers.

We all have different General Adaptive Potentials; each of us responds to stressors in different ways. Some of us may handle mental stress better than others while some might do better with physical stress. Some people may develop lung cancer after just a few cigarettes while some people might seem ok. Some people get digestive distress from a little bit of sugar while others seem to handle it ok.

Both cigarettes and sugar are stressors and just because you don't feel anything wrong does not mean your mind-body is not having to compensate, adapt and defend against what you're exposing it to.

How long does it take? How imbalanced are you?

There is no process in the universe that does not take time and the same is true for real, meaningful regeneration of your mind-body.

The more your mind-body is showing signs of defence and decay, the more time and attention you'll need for growth and repair. This will frustrate you because the more your mind-body is imbalanced the more desperate you are for fast relief.

If what you really want is a bigger life, if you really want to look good naked, feel good about how you look, express energy, have focus and Thrive!, then you are going to have to give yourself some time and attention. While most people will begin to notice differences within the first few weeks, about 20% won't. This 20% needs to work harder than the 80%. The 20% needs to be more patient than the 80%. You are not broken; you are just a seed that needs a little more attention and a little more time for you to bloom.

We need to address all three dimensions of lifestyle to maximise nutrients and minimise stressors. Many times we eat well and move well, but unless we are thinking well some of us might not see the change we want.

Be patient with your mind-body and know that it is intelligently dealing with the scars of your stressors and is adapting the best it can. Also know that it is grateful for all the nutrients you are now feeding it. Your cells are revelling in each rock that you unpack from your backpack.

Be kind to your mind-body and allow it to intelligently marshal that orchestra of vitality. Feed it nutrients and listen carefully as it starts to produce more wonderful melodies as you experience more up days and fewer down days. Each rock you unpack now is an investment in your human potential, your personal performance. The more you unpack the more return you will get on your investment.

Pay attention to your mind-body and cultivate awareness so that you can notice the changes that happen. Sometimes children are so busy looking for the roots to appear from their seed that they completely miss the leaves! Some of us get so bogged down watching our weight that we don't notice that our energy has improved or our skin looks better or that we're smiling more. There is nothing bigger than the little things. Changes are going to happen, not necessarily in the order that you'd like but certainly in the order that your mind-body needs.

A special note on fat loss
To lose fat you have to allow your mind-body to shed the excess insulation. Your mind-body has gained this fat in response to stressors in your past and now, by providing nutrients, you can allow it to intelligently let it go.

Some people will lose fat quickly while others will lose it slowly. Some beans grow quickly and some grow a little slower. Your mind-body might need some extra time and attention; you might have to be a little more rigid in your eating, moving and thinking than others. Make peace with this fact and move on; don't allow what the scale tells you to become an additional stressor to hold you back.

In fact the bathroom scale or even the scale in your doctor's room can be very misleading. Muscle weighs more than fat, so if you're losing fat but gaining muscle then the scale might tell you that you are staying the same weight or even getting a little heavier.

The bathroom scale can breed neurosis in another way, too. I've heard of people reporting weight going up and down by as much as 3 and even 4kg in a day. This can be affected by fluctuation in hormone levels, how much salt or carbohydrates you've eaten, your degree of hydration and what kind of training you're doing and many other factors.

More meaningful than the scale is the tape measure to measure your waist line. The amount of belly fat we have is a very strong and important indicator about our level of health. Another way to judge your fat loss is by the fit of your clothes.

All 3 stressors
I recently heard about a man who went kayaking on the sea with friends. He was known to be fit and strong. They all headed out from to a buoy and had turned around to head back to shore when they noticed he wasn't with them anymore.

A surf rescue team found him later still paddling straight out to sea but he was otherwise completely unresponsive. He was taken to hospital and tests showed he had a cancerous tumour pressing on his brain and he was dead within a week.

The next time you or someone around you complains that their friend can eat whatever he likes and not put on weight, gently remind them that what they put into their body will always affect the balance of their ecosystem. Health problems don't always show from the outside and can take decades to develop.

As many as 40% of people with normal body weight will suffer from metabolic abnormalities typically associated with obesity, including high blood pressure, unbalanced cholesterol levels, non-alcoholic fatty liver disease, and cardiovascular disease. Some imbalances show on the outside and some don't, but just because it does not show it doesn't mean there isn't damage being done.

Researchers have coined the term TOFI for just such a person. TOFI stands for 'thin outside fat inside' and it is given to a person who looks normal or skinny from the outside but under an MRI scanner shows a significant amount of internal fat. This is the 'skinny fat person' who has a normal to slim waist line but a significant and harmful layer of fat around their internal organs. This internal fat seems to be the most dangerous type. It can be thought of as an organ that is constantly leaking chronic inflammation, defence and decay, signalling to your brain that you are still hungry, causing you to overeat. Remember that with prolonged exposure chronic inflammation shrinks your brain, shreds your arteries, demineralises your bones, cannibalises your muscles, imbalances your hormones, punch holes in your gut and weakens your immune system. ●

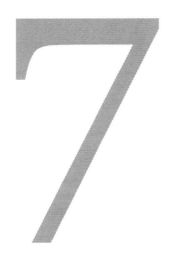

The art and science of change

Your blindspot.
Why you'll fail.
You crave meaning.
The genesis of health.
The 4 Lenses for transformation.
A good starting point.

Why you've failed before and how you can learn to transform?

> *Insanity is doing the same thing over and over again*
> *and expecting different results.*
> ALBERT EINSTEIN

In an often quoted study from Illinois in the USA, that compared people who had won the lottery with people who suffered trauma resulting in paralysis, researchers wanted to find out who was happier one year after the event: lottery winners or paraplegics? I thought that the answer would be easy: lottery winners would be more content, right?

What came out of the study was truly surprising. When the researchers looked at the scores for future expected happiness and how much pleasure the subjects took out of everyday activities, both groups were about the same. The lottery winners experienced a period of elation following their windfall, but often had setbacks affecting their mental well-being. Many of them had as much or less money than they started with.

Paraplegic trauma victims, however, usually went through a period of depression but their state of mental well-being often stabilised.

Doesn't this sound suspiciously like our lives right now? No matter how much we try, we don't seem to shift the needle on happiness or fulfilment on our weight or our levels of energy and focus beyond just a few weeks or months.

Thoughts and choices flow like a stream
A drop of water glides over a smooth stone, making a small and imperceptible groove as it moves. The next drop of water follows the small groove and runs along it, too. Then, as more and more drops fall and follow the groove, each drop makes the groove slightly larger.

Over many years, with millions and millions of drops of water, the groove becomes a gully, the gully becomes a ravine, the ravine becomes a gorge and the gorge becomes a canyon. Now a drop of water falling on the original spot is compelled by the immutable law of gravity to follow the same course as the original drop. It follows the path of least resistance and it will take some monumental force of nature like a flood or an earthquake to change the course of the river. Without that flood or earthquake the river continues to run as it always has.

The neurones in our brains show us how we make choices. If we were to start with a blank slate we could make any choice we wanted with ease. The choices we make every day, however, make a groove and, choice by choice, day by day we've worn ravines of habits that have then been carved into our nervous system like canyons. To make new choices over a prolonged period of time can be incredibly difficult and this is proven by the legions of us who have tried diets and lost weight only to regain it a short while later.

Thoughts and feelings that become decisions are sparks that fire along nerves in our brain. Each time a spark fires along nerves it links them, lightly at first, making it easier for the spark to ignite the same nerve pathway again – it's called neuroplasticity. As it follows the same nerve path over and over again the link between the nerves gets stronger and stronger. Scientists have coined the phrase 'Nerves that fire together, wire together.'

For the drop of water following the course of the river, once it's in the canyon, there is no chance of it changing the course of the river. The best chance we have of helping the drop to take a new path is to change its course at the start, and help it carve a new groove.

The same is true for our habits and behaviour: they are grooved into our brain by well fired and wired nerve pathways that are tough to change. But if we can look to the source, like the drop of water, then we have the best chance of making a sustainable change.

The anatomy of a transformation

We know we need to change, that much is clear. We need to change the way we eat, the way we move and the way we think. If diets fail, exercise doesn't last and positive thinking is a sham; what can we do? If conventional wisdom has become conventional confusion, what are we to think?

Let's get back to basics. Let's not treat the symptom by trying a new diet; let's find out why diets fail. Let's not go down the same well-worn path and hope that it will be different this time: it won't! Let's do something new by looking upstream to find the source of the problem.

We know the results you get in your life are a function of your behaviour and the choices you make every day. To get results we need to act.

Our actions and behaviours are themselves governed by something higher. Marketers have known for years that the choices we make and the action we take are not always rational. Our buying decisions, like all decisions, are not governed by our higher cognitive areas, as much as we would like to believe they are. Our rational mind is hardly ever in control of the thousands of small and large choices, decisions and judgements we make. Rather it is our emotions that guide our behaviour and our habits.

You've heard the term emotional eating but might not know that this doesn't just apply to finishing that tub of ice cream when we're feeling low. All eating is emotional because what you've chosen to eat was guided by an emotion, a feeling. Your state of mind is also a result of the emotions you experience. Whether you feel stressed or you feel calm, they are *feelings* just like happiness and sadness. Whether you engage in some physical activity today either in the gym or outside is also a direct result of how you *feel* about it.

So unless we're addressing emotions, we're not even scratching the surface. Herein lies the truth about most diet, exercise or self-improvement systems. Their marketing influences your emotions by helping you to buy, buy, buy, based on how they make you feel. Very few of them then use that same principle to get you emotionally engaged in the change they are asking you to make. This is why your 'change' doesn't last long.

Emotions are important but we are not yet at the source. The source lies even higher up in the hierarchy of human behaviour. The source lies with your values and beliefs, what you could call your philosophy of life.

Here at the summit of human behaviour we are at the point where thoughts, emotions, actions, behaviours, habits, results and ultimately our quality of life emanates from. It is right here that we can influence which way that drop of water goes, which nerve pathway a spark lights up.

Long term habits are hard to change because they are walled into a canyon driven by our emotions. By becoming aware of and shifting your philosophy of life, you can avoid the old canyon all together and create something new, something better.

126

At this point you can move beyond change and begin to truly transform. This is where Thrive! starts: at the source.

What do I need to do to begin to change?

> *People will choose unhappiness over uncertainty.*
> TIM FERRISS

We are creatures of habit and there is a good reason for that. We are only able to use so much cognitive function a day and if we can automate a lot of what we do that is repetitive day in and day out, then that process frees our brain power to concentrate on the new and novel things that come our way.

Imagine how hard it would be to drive a car if you had to constantly concentrate on changing gears and working the pedals. What we do really well is learn something new and then make it routine.

Just like changing the gears on a car can become automatic, so can the way we think and behave.

One problem with routine is that it can be hard to change. Some people find it near impossible to change their patterns of thought and behaviour. Meet them when they're in their 50's and they are often in the same pattern of thought that they were in their 20's.

Our current lifestyle habits are robbing us of our true potential, making us live our lives of quiet desperation in fuzzy sepia while missing out on the High Definition world that we could exist in.

Routine can often bring us a promise of comfort and security but does it always deliver? An alcoholic or an addict could be in a routine that is destructive and yet they fail to acknowledge their illness. For whatever reason, they are comfortable enough in their cocoon of self-deception to resist changing their condition. Others may be able to see their self-destructive habits, but the alcoholic or addict still refuses to admit it to themselves. It is their intense discomfort and insecurity with their deeper selves that drives their evasive behaviour, yet it provides a superficial comfort and security all of its own.

Some of our habits and patterns, while not as extreme as a needle-using junkie, are probably also destructive but we don't see it that way. Maybe we eat too much sugar or don't exercise enough; maybe we are holding onto resentment or guilt. These are patterns of behaviour, routines that we carry around with us whether we like it or not. Since it's on the inside, like a junkie looking for a fix we might not see the damage we're doing, but it's essential that you open your heart and mind and examine your lifestyle in a new and honest light.

Some people say that an addict has to hit 'rock bottom' before they will really make a change. They will hit a point so low in their lives that they will have to look in the mirror and face some hard truths that will then catalyse their rehabilitation. 'Rock bottom' is the point at which a person is forced to face their deepest values and beliefs. Who am I? Why am I here? What kind of person am I? This is their philosophy of life and it is the source from which their thoughts, emotions and actions flow.

This is the veritable earthquake that disturbs the flow of the river so that it can break free of its canyon and forge a new path to a new destiny. This is one path to transformation.

Realisation does not mean having to reach 'rock bottom'; there is another way. The turning point where transformation becomes more likely is any time at which you go upstream to the source, when you face up to your philosophy of life. This is when you realise that the pain of staying the same is more than the pain of changing. When you have suffered enough to ask the hard questions of yourself then you don't just change, you transform.

How do I make change comfortable, effective and sustainable?

When the why is big enough, the how takes care of itself.
JIM ROHN

To be able to make the kind change that you're looking for: change that has real benefits beyond the superficial; change that sticks beyond the next fad and change that is manageable because it is comfortably uncomfortable, you need more than change. You need transformation and to transform you need to address your inner "Why."

Your "Why" is your highest value, the things that matter most to you, the areas in your life where you are most organised, disciplined and resourceful. These values are different for each of us, they are uniquely ours and because of that only we can find out what they are. Your values are the fundamental thing that makes you tick. Knowing your values becomes meaningful, and meaningful change is transformation.

These values give your life meaning and they move you and can make you move mountains. Anytime a person is pushed to go beyond their self-imposed limitations to do something extraordinary it's because their values were driving them there. You can tap into that kind of drive, that power of will. You have it within you to move mountains and we will be guiding you to the source of that power.

For you to make effective change you have to know where you are now; you have to know what your values are. The problem is that, for most of us, our values lie in our subconscious. They operate in the shadowy background just as the coding of an operating system runs a computer. What you need to do is to shine a light on your values and the best way to do that is to find out what values your life demonstrates. That means that by looking at the past and searching for patterns you will gain a much better understanding of what your values are and how you have been operating.

Next we'll be giving you real life tools and techniques that make change more manageable; this is the "How": how to plan change, how to track change, how to measure change. These tools make change a game instead of a drag, a challenge instead of a slog. This is what makes change understandable.

The final piece of the puzzle is the "What": the on the ground, day to day of what to eat, what movement to do and what kind of thought patterns make changes stick. This is what makes change manageable; what you are going to be doing on a daily basis as you form new habits.

When we talk about this you'll realise even more that this is no ordinary 'diet and exercise' book. This is a revelation. We're going to go against the grain and will probably contradict most other advice that you've gotten before. We have delved into the science of wellness and realised that most diet and exercise information is misguided and very limited in its scope, and so gets very limited results.

Put down the pills, get off the treadmill, ditch the low-fat foods, throw away your whole grains, stop trying to 'think positively'; time to shift from 'weights and cardio' to something much more exciting. You're in for a few surprises.

The neurology of change

"I want vitality, now what?"

It's been said that to change our lives we need to change our habits and while that's true it's not the whole truth. We truly are creatures of habit and your habits determine your destiny. Changing your habits will help you to move toward a new destiny, where you can Thrive! in *vitality* and live a bigger and better Life.

The problem is that changing your habits is hard. Only 10% of heart bypass patients address the damage their lifestyle has created and sustain these changes past the first two post-operative years. So if someone is not changed by the stark reality of heart surgery, then what chance do you have?

There is a flow to making real, sustainable change that can help you to live the life you've been looking for. By understanding this flow you can discover the truth and make change that is comfortable, sustainable and effective – that is more than just change: it's transformation.

I've used this flow for myself and my family and I've used it for people in my practice and the people I coach. Countless people who have learned this science of change have used it, too, and it works.

The people in the Lottery Winner and Trauma Victim study (see page 124) are simply returning to the set point for happiness and pleasure that had been grooved in their mind and brain before their respective life-changing events. Just like those participants you have a deeply ingrained set of values and beliefs that drive your emotions, habits and give you the results you see in life.

Over the course of your lifetime, this deep ingraining of neural pathways has produced a set-point: your levels of health, happiness, wealth and success that you have and are likely to continue to have for the rest of your life. Much like the course of a river in a canyon, these patterns are so deeply engrained that they are very tough to try and change.

Why the "Why" is so important

In the quest for lifelong vitality and finding the headspace that allows us to get there we have several good models to guide us. Salutogenesis – Latin, *sales* for health and *genesis* for origin – is one which has had profound implications in health care. Instead of focusing on the cause of disease it focuses on improving and maintaining health.

According to this model, when in a state of coherence, a person is likely to live longer, enjoy a good quality of life and enjoy good mental and physical well-being. You could say that such a person is dancing through the chaos of life. In a state of coherence, your degree of personal confidence is high, your life and its demands are meaningful and you feel you have the resources to meets life's challenges: you are able to change, adapt and Thrive!

Aaron Antonovsky who first coined the term salutogenesis and wrote two books on the subject, found that 29% of women who survived the concentration camps of World War II still had positive emotional health. In the face of unimaginable cruelty and suffering, these women still managed to reconcile their experience without debilitating emotional scars because they had a sense of coherence: the ability to change, adapt and thrive amid significant stressors.

Antonovsky found that a sense of coherence predicts better well-being in all areas of life despite stressful situations and severe hardships. Salutogenesis has been tested and validated in many fields including medicine, psychiatry, health psychology and behavioural and preventative medicine.

Antonovsky described and tested three components to being in a state of coherence:
* **Meaningfulness** – the belief that things in your life make sense emotionally and are source of fulfilment.
* **Manageability** – the belief that you have the ability and resources to meet the demands you may face.
* **Comprehensibility** – the belief that things that confront you are able to be understood.

If we apply these components to the world of lifestyle change and personal growth we can convert them into three questions, and if we can answer all three then we will move towards a state of personal coherence.

- WHY – this is about purpose. Why will making change to your lifestyle help you to lead a more *meaningful* life, one that brings purpose? Why will changing be worthwhile to you?
- HOW – this is about strategy. How will you *comprehend* the challenge and effectively accumulate and deploy the resources necessary to get through and sustain the change?
- WHAT – this is about tactics. What will you do – and in what order – to make your life reasonably predicable and *manageable*?

To make change effective, sustainable and comfortable, you need three things: purpose, strategy and tactics. Of the three, purpose is the most significant and without it strategy and tactics matter very little.

Without the "Why" you've got no reason to take any action and any action you might take will be purposeless, misguided or just plain random. With a strong sense of purpose, however, you can begin to critically assess your strategies and tactics to find the ones that work for you. You can begin to refine your transformation with focus and drive and improve your chances of success.

After successive failures in the Rugby World Cup and a heavy defeat to South Africa in 2004 the All Blacks, arguably the most successful sports franchise in the world, were in trouble. The night they lost heavily to South Africa and finished last in the annual Tri-Nations rugby tournament, many of their team were so drunk that they were found passed out in the corridors and bushes of their hotel. Some were so drunk that their teammates feared their lives were at risk. Poor results, players, mangers and coaches threatening to leave and social dysfunction – this was not the demeanour of world class professionals.

After a long flight back to Wellington 8 members of management and senior players sat in a room and had a meeting that lasted 3 days. The question they had to answer before leaving was 'Why?' Why did they play rugby, why was the All Black institution different? They were searching for a new purpose.

The redefinition of that purpose lead to a complete overhaul for the All Blacks. The management structure changed, practice techniques changed, their ethics and code of conduct changed, their haka (the war cry they perform before matches) even changed and, with time, so did their results. The records show that the All Blacks have made themselves even more successful. Their win ratio from 2011 to

2015 was 91%, they are the only team to have won two consecutive World Cups and have now won three in total.

BE – DO – HAVE

Be – Do – Have is another model of human behaviour that provides a map, guiding us though this terrain of transformation.

This model tells us – for example – that the results of *having* more money is more likely to be a result of what we *do* consistently, like earn and invest wisely. The *have* depends on the *do*.

What we regularly *do*, like saving and investing, is a result of our state of *being*. Some people tend to be spenders and others savers; some are producers and others are consumers. The *do* depends on the *be*.

Therefore what you *have* will always be aligned with what you *do* which will always reflect your state of *being*. Be – Do – Have.

The people who won the lottery didn't necessarily do the things that attract long term wealth because they hadn't become the type of person with such a habit. They weren't *being* wealthy people and so weren't *doing* the things that would have caused them to *have* lasting riches.

What they had was good fortune that sent manna from heaven in the form of the lottery. The study tells us that most of the winners didn't seem to change their behaviour very much and spent more than they invested and consumed more than they produced. They carried out this destructive behaviour because there was no change in their values and beliefs concerning money, and so their actions whittled away at their lottery winnings until they were roughly back to where they had started.

They had violated the Be – Do – Have model. Since they hadn't made shifts upstream in their *being*, their *doing* corrected back to a set point of *having*. That set point is governed by your innermost beliefs about yourself and your world, how those beliefs drive your emotions, your behaviour and your results.

This principle holds true for the paraplegic group, too. Following severe trauma and a diagnosis of lifelong handicap their happiness levels also returned to their set point.

Increased energy, weight management, mental clarity, focus and attention, physical health and vitality and resistance to disease are all results of Be – Do – Have . They are all part of the *have*. They depend on what we *do* and that depends on our state of *being*.

Your weight, your happiness, your levels of energy, your strength and your focus in life are all governed by your internal set point, your state of *being*. Put simply it's the sum total of who you are. To transform you have to alter some part of who you are. This may sound scary, even impossible, but all you'll be doing is revealing what's underneath, your true self, and then letting that shine.

WHY – HOW – WHAT

As you read this there is something that you know you could be doing to make yourself healthier or happier, but you're not doing it. You know of a way you could be eating less of this or more of that, getting up earlier in the morning, doing more exercise or any number of small things that would make you more content and get you into better shape; but you're not. This isn't because you're lazy, it's not because you're bad.

You know some of the *what* to do, in fact I think you've probably been so inundated with directions of what to do that you've become paralysed by doubt. Eat high fat, eat low fat, eat high carb, eat low carb, do a detox, do a soup diet, do a juice diet, eat meat, be a vegan... it becomes just too much and so you end up doing nothing.

Virtually all diets and exercise programs currently available are short term patch-ups and not lifestyle solutions. They might help to produce some change for a while, but they don't seem to last, do they? No wonder we become so cynical about diets and so, instead of being disappointed by trying something new, we simply keep doing what we've always done.

A lot of the time, knowing *what* to do isn't the biggest issue; the issue is knowing *how* to do it. How do you choose which option is the right one for you? How do you make that option work?

When you know *how* you're going to make change in your life things seems easier, more achievable. Like having a map, you can plan for kinks in the road and you can be prepared for challenging situations. Your map gives you an idea of what to expect next. It gives you the time to formulate a plan of action to achieve what you want.

If you're going to change the way you eat you can clear your kitchen cupboards of all the foods you need to avoid. You can create meal plans and shopping lists to help you have at hand the kinds of food you need. You can ask a friend or significant other to be an accountability partner, making sure you're doing the things you have committed to.

If you're going to change the way you move you can plan your workout or a running route in advance. Join a group or a club that are doing the same thing, whether a CrossFit gym or a running club. Being with other people makes change easier. These are your tactics for improving your probability of success, much like the tactics a football team employs when they go into a game. The players know *what* they need to do (score goals) but knowing *how* they are going to do it is vital. Are they going to grind away at the opposition, go down the flanks or hit them on the counter attack? These are the decisions that will decide whether they win, lose or draw any given game.

If the *how* is like having a map that helps us know *what* to do then the *why* is the question that picks your destination. Before you leave your home each morning you get dressed, *why* you're leaving the house sets the tone for the *what* and the *how* of your preparations for the day ahead. Got an important meeting? Well then, how you get ready and what you wear will be very different to going out for a run.

A "WHY" CASE HISTORY:

Lisa, a coaching client came to me saying that she wanted to lose weight. When I asked her why she crossed her arms, looked at me quizzically and said that it was obvious that she was overweight and wanted to look good again. I explained the importance of *why* and how vital it is to the process of making a change like losing weight.

Initially she was adamant that her desire for the change was just to look good. As we delved deeper she realised that she wanted to look good to feel comfortable in a bikini again, because summer was coming.

More discussion revealed that she wanted to feel comfortable in her bikini again because she wanted to be able to get out and be more active.

Reason after reason, deeper and deeper, we unravelled what was the core issue of her desire to lose weight: Lisa's desire to attract the right life partner, and preparing her body to carry, deliver and raise healthy children.

So when she first came in she was asking me about fat burning pills and meal replacement formulas because she thought she was looking for a shortcut and by the end she was convinced she needed to reassess how she was eating, moving and thinking.

Why is the question that gets it all started.

Why is the most important question you can ask.

Why is the question that will begin to shine a light on your values and beliefs.

The deeper you go into your *why*, the clearer your path becomes. The clearer your path, the easier the journey.

Guiding Why

To help you find your Guiding Why, I've created a free resource that will help you identify and clarify your highest life values: what are the things that drive you; what is your meaning in life?

Visit http://THRIVElifestyle.solutions/why

Why the "How" is so important

When you ask *how*, you're asking for a strategy. You're asking for a plan of attack. What you want out of this is the knowledge that you have the resources you need and the ability to use those resources on your journey to vitality.

Carol Dweck, PhD is a professor of psychology, author of several books and a researcher who has studied motivation and behaviour at Stanford University for nearly forty years. Her work has revealed a powerful insight: what people believe shapes what they achieve. How you approach a challenge is much more important than how talented, intelligent or able you are.

Already, as you read this book, you are considering *how* you could apply these tools to changing your life, and whether this is going to work for you. There are two ways you can answer this question:

The first it to look for *impossibility* – you will look for and find reasons why this won't work for you because you probably started reading the book with this mindset. You might already have found some seemingly valid reasons why you can't take the time to find your Guiding Why. Maybe you told yourself that you'll get to it later or you can't afford the time. Put simply, you have already found impossibility.

The alternative is to look for *possibility*, and approach the changes that you want in your life with a sense of adventure. Nothing is being forced on you. Your desire for change is your choice and is in your hands: only you can make it possible.

Asking *whether* this is going to work for you is the wrong question. Asking *how* this is going to work for you will put you on track for possibility.

We're going to help with some resources to make things as easy as possible and to make implementation simpler, but the truth is the buck stops with your mindset; it is your ultimate resource.

When my daughter was just under two and toddling everywhere I loved watching her explore the world. Have you ever noticed how, before kids get programmed by society, they can be almost fearless in the face of new things? She went into new places, spaces and situations and approached new things with an open sense of curiosity and play. She shrieked and smiled as she experienced and discovered this new world. Sometimes she got hurt or scared by something new, but as long as she felt safe and secure she'd get right up and try again before the tears on her cheeks had even dried.

Playfulness and curiosity are the cornerstones of learning and growth in life. When you're playful then mistakes aren't a personal failing. When you're curious and trying something new that doesn't work out it doesn't make you wrong, it's just another bit of information that helps you figure out what will work.

I have failed often and I still fail and I will fail in the future. I fail a lot. I'm wrong a lot. It is a natural part of my learning journey. When you've stopped failing then you've stopped growing. In our practice and in my home we often tell each other about what we've failed at during the day. This opens each of us to the concept of continued personal growth with honesty about our challenges so that we can find solutions. It helps us to look for *possibility* and not to get stuck in *impossibility*.

IMPOSSIBILITY:
I can't go online and complete my Guiding Why now because: I'm too busy/ it's too late/ it won't work anyway/ I can do this without help.

POSSIBILTY:
I can schedule 10 minutes in for tomorrow/ let's see if this thing works/ let's see how much I can learn.

Visit http://THRIVElifestyle.solutions/why

Have skin in the game

If you've ever played poker you know about the concept that you have to pay to play. In competitive matches there are no free rides, you have to have skin in the game. Sometimes in poker one person wins the pot because everyone else has folded. The winner usually doesn't have to show his cards because everyone else has quit. When I first experienced this I couldn't believe that we would all just let this guy take our money and not see his cards. A friend who introduced me to the game just said, "You have to pay to see their cards." What he meant was that I had to be willing to match or raise the winner's bet to see his cards.

The same applies to lifestyle transformation; you have to be willing to commit to the process to be able to have the best chance of getting good results.

Having something to lose makes us committed to win. In studies where they test the emotional charge of winning or losing the answer is very clear: we hate losing. We hate losing R100 more than we love winning R100. We hate losing out on personal pride when we don't do what we said we would do. We hate knowing that other people know that we failed, even if they don't care. Public failures hurt more than private ones do.

Now that you're looking for *possibility*, you need to make a small but open commitment to have some skin in the game. You can make your commitment to *possibility* to just a few trusted supporters or you can make it online to a group of people who love and support you. By doing this openly you are not only affirming that you are committed to making change you are also more likely to succeed.

4 Lenses

While practicing, coaching and in my online lifestyle mastery programs I have not only witnessed many extraordinary transformations but also many missed opportunities. Many people give up on the verge of breakthroughs.

This experience led me to research and develop a 4 lens model to help people change the way they view their journey. Carol Dweck advocates that it is the way in which we frame our change and our efforts that will make a massive difference between hitting the bullseye or scoring a near miss.

LENS 1:   Begin with the end in mind

> *If you don't know where you are going, you'll end up some place else.*
> YOGI BERRA

When you're looking to create transformation it is important to know what you're aiming for. This 'end in mind' is your *Guiding Why*, it's your purpose and it's the first lens for creating transformation.

LENS 2:   What's my next step

> *Even the longest of journeys begins with a single step.*
> LAOZI IN THE TAO TE CHING

Once you have your purpose in place you can break up your journey into manageable chunks. If your plan is to run a marathon and you can't walk around the block then it would be unwise to attempt the full 42km from the beginning. Instead it would be useful to aim to walk around the block, then run round the block and then increase your running distance over time.

When we try to look at the whole without breaking it into chunks we can get overwhelmed and frustrated by our lack of progress. When you have the end in mind, and you measure your progress on your next goal, life becomes a lot easier.

LENS 3: Carve your own path

> *You can't connect the dots looking forward;*
> *you can only connect them looking backwards.*
> *So you have to trust that the dots will somehow connect in your future.*
> STEVE JOBS

Despite your best efforts, your path from A to B is never going to be a straight line. You will meander and there is richness and learning in your individual journey. Embrace that.

Your transformation is going to be different to anyone else's and judging your progress based on someone else's map is not useful. You are master of your own ship, you are in charge and the things you need to learn on your journey are uniquely yours. Trust in your own journey.

LENS 4: No failure only feedback

> *I've missed more than 9000 shots in my career. I've lost almost 300 games.*
> *26 times, I've been trusted to take the game winning shot and missed.*
> *I've failed over and over and over again in my life. And that is why I succeed.*
> MICHAEL JORDAN

The Japanese principle of *Kaizen* is one of constant refinement and improvement. This is useful in those moments where you might have fallen off the wagon or strayed from your plan. We call it going offroad.

Instead of viewing it as a failure, view it as a learning experience. Instead of berating yourself for your weak will power, take a moment to reflect on your choices and learn how you could do better next time.

If you embark on a new nutritional plan that excludes certain foods, it's only human nature that you will then want those foods. In the face of wanting that which is forbidden, your willpower does not last very long and it takes a lot of energy to sustain. When you do eventually succumb, which we all do, you feel guilt, shame and frustration and those emotions often lead us to give up completely.

The offroad moments are inevitable and can be very useful so why not harness part of human nature and plan them? Bypass the willpower and guilt all together by planning your offroad moments about once a week to once a month depending on your allostatic load. The planned one day of eating poorly is better than the one week unscheduled binge. Making these offroad moments part of the plan minimises your chances of feeling like a complete failure and maximises your chances of getting back on track.

Ditch the guilt. If it's chocolate cake that threatens to break your willpower then allow yourself an offroad excursion periodically and enjoy every bite. Savour the flavour without feeling bad about it and know that you will do better tomorrow.

Using this lens you embrace 'failure' because you realise it's part of the process and makes you stronger. Over time as you get back on track after your offroad moments you'll notice that they happen less and less, and you don't crave that which you can't have as much anymore.

What is the "What"

N ow we can focus on basic tactics: the things you will do every day to make your changes – no matter how small – add up to a transformation.

The reality of most self-help, diet and exercise books that line the shelves of your local book store or even your bookcase, is that most of them aren't read and if they are, the advice they offer isn't implemented. So, while diet and exercise are lucrative subject matter for book sales it's the least meaningful: it's what everyone wants to know but no one wants to do.

This does not mean it's not important. Having the small details worked out for you is obviously useful but it's more useful if done in the context of the larger mission.

When the "Why" is big enough, the "How" and the "What" will sort themselves out. This means that in those moments when you feel stuck and frustrated, when you feel like a failure, this is the best time to revisit your 'Guiding Why', your purpose and to refocus on the higher, more meaningful goal.

Such moments of confusion, frustration and feeling like a failure are essential. These states of confusion pre-empt your next breakthrough. Most of us have never been given the tools to understand this process because we've never been asked about the "Why" and the "How". We don't see these momentary doubts as a prelude to success, we see them as failure. The difference between failure and breakthrough is whether your "Why" is big enough to keep you moving on.

The difference between people who give up and those that breakthrough is that those who breakthrough get up again and continue with renewed energy and focus. They don't use a temporary setback as an excuse to undo all the good they have achieved. They ask new questions and try new answers and keep going until it works. It's the stories we tell ourselves that make the difference. Excuses simply turn a temporary setback into a failure.

Randy Pauch was a lecturer with terminal cancer. Before he died he created a Last Lecture for his children and then shared this gift with the world. He was featured on Oprah and had his Last Lecture published as a book.

One of Randy's lessons was that 'walls' only exist to keep out those who don't *really* want what is beyond the wall. Climbing over a wall allows you to prove to yourself that you want what's there badly enough to do whatever it takes to breakthrough.

Just doing the "What" on its own is not enough. Doing the "What" without knowing the "Why" or the "How" will damage the process of your transformation. For this reason we have the information on nutrition, movement and headspace in the last section of the book. ●

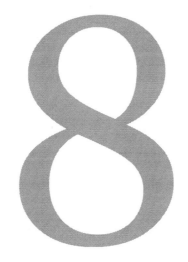

Activate your
wellness genes

The genius in your genes.
Freeing a domesticated human.
Pornography, the weakness in your genes.

How do we create vitality?

Y ou are an intelligent ecosystem, complex and organised. You also know that, as an animal, you have evolved to expect certain biologically appropriate signals to activate genes that produce growth and repair. Those signals come through purity and sufficiency of chemical, physical and mental factors in your lifestyle – in other words, the way you eat, move, think, rest, experience nature and breathe. These are nutrients.

Along with these nutrients you need alignment of your spine so your nervous system can send and receive nerve signals to every cell in your body without interference. Feed your mind-body nutrients and realign it, and you then activate your genes for growth and repair. Given good alignment, enough nutrients and enough time you will move toward vitality and really begin to Thrive!

When you are toxic or deficient in your lifestyle or have poor alignment then you are in a state of dis-ease and are giving your genes the signals that they must defend. If you continue to expose your mind-body to stressors and misalignment then your defence eventually gives way to decay and disease.

In your day-to-day life, one stressor does not cause a disease but it does switch your system into defence mode. The accumulation of stressors over time leaves indelible scars. This is when short term defence turns into long term decay. You can adapt in a state of defence, but only for so long before you succumb to fatigue and defence becomes decay.

Each time you choose to eat, move, think rest, get into nature or breath in ways that are incompatible with your genetic code and every moment you live with misalignment of your spine you forfeit some of your life's potential. Your ability to live a bigger life rests on the amount of growth and repair you are expressing. The longer we live with adaptation and compensation, the longer it takes to undo. The deeper the dysfunction is buried, the longer it takes to uncover.

Unpack the backpack
Just as the accumulation of stressors over time can damage us, so too can the accumulation of nutrients over time help us regenerate. We have layered on the problems, so we need to layer on the solutions, one at a time. Choosing to unload even the smallest of stressors from your allostatic backpack begins to move you in

the direction of growth and repair. When you make it a habit to unload stressors and take on nutrients and to realign your spine, then you accelerate the process as each action builds on the one before it. Now you are building momentum and the more you build the easier it gets.

What do we model this on?

When you're searching for what you need to do to minimise stressors and maximise resistance it pays to look to biology to figure out what makes a stressor and a nutrient. A stressor for one animal may be a nutrient to another.

100% dark chocolate used in cooking can be delicious. It's bitter but if you use just enough on the right dish you can delight your senses. That dark chocolate is also packed with antioxidants and a compound called theobromine. Theobromine in small doses can have a positive anti-inflammatory effect for people with chronic pain and inflammation. Theobromine in dogs, however, is highly toxic and can even kill them.

In Madagascar, one species of lemur, the Gentle Bamboo Lemur, eats the stem of a certain type of bamboo but avoids the shoots because they contain a high concentration of cyanide. Another species, the Golden Bamboo Lemur, which was only discovered in 1984, making it the world's most recently discovered primate, has no such qualms. The Golden Bamboo Lemur can eat 12 times the fatal dose of cyanide held in the bamboo shoot and thrive. No one knows how the Golden Bamboo Lemur does it but it shows us that one animal's food is another's toxin.

These examples show us that nutrients and toxins in all forms – chemical, mental and physical – are biologically specific for different species of animals. Nutrients are biologically appropriate, while stressors are biologically inappropriate.

Wild, free humans provide us with a template of what is biologically appropriate for us, homo sapiens sapiens. They give us a framework of thought and enquiry from which to discover what our genes expect for vitality.

Modern health science is still young and doesn't have a broad appreciation of the human being and its place in nature. This is why we still have so many contradictory opinions, and more questions than answers. It's like the old story of blind men examining an elephant, each trying to describing what they are feeling.

The blind man at the front thinks he's got his hands on a thick, rubbery hose. Another thinks he's feeling a broad floppy fan while another thinks he's embracing a wide rough pillar. They are all accurate in their individual interpretations but they are missing the bigger picture – they are feeling parts of an elephant! The first man felt the trunk, the second had an ear and the last had a leg.

The bigger picture for you is not weight-loss, though that's obviously part of it. The bigger picture is not treating specific conditions or diseases, though that's also part of it. The bigger picture is helping your mind-body to do what it intelligently does best: grow and repair to help you experience vitality so you can Thrive!

Out of the complexity of all the health research that exists and the many opinions that you hear, there is an elegantly simple approach: by defining your premise you can begin to find that simplicity beyond the complexity, to see the bigger picture and to start to fill in the details.

The domesticated human
The bigger picture is realising that we humans are animals; we are a part of nature and we have domesticated ourselves. In our human zoo we have devised a completely artificial lifestyle, including our nutrition, movement and headspace, and this is hurting us.

By creating a 'biologically appropriate' lifestyle we can rediscover our innate potential for vitality. We can give our mind-body the nourishment it needs to be able to gain energy, shed excess fat, resist disease, clear the mind, find focus, get fit for life and get our lives back.

The wild, free human
Since each animal in the wild has evolved to match their genes to the environment, what we call the evolutionary sweet spot, we can use wild animals as guides to help us find what is biologically appropriate for humans.

Just like Mokolo's zoo keepers used data on wild, free gorillas to find out what he should be eating, what his enclosure should look like and what temperature it should be, so too can we look to wild free humans to give us a template for our lifestyle.

By looking at what wild, free humans did we get an idea of what is and what is not biologically appropriate for us. They give us very good clues as to what purity and sufficiency looks like, and what toxicity and deficiency in human beings looks like.

Why use them?

You may have heard of the Paleo Diet or the Primal Blueprint, which some refer to as a primal or ancestral lifestyle. This approach says that we lived as hunter-gatherers for more than 90% of our existence and that the rapid changes to our surroundings have put us at odds with what our genes expect. This evolutionary template has become quite popular, but also widely misinterpreted.

Mark Sisson, author of the *Primal Blueprint and the Primal Connection* and godfather of the primal/paleo/ancestral health movement cites research that indicates our wild, free humans lived lives of incredible affluence. Affluence here does not mean rich in money terms, but rich in terms of options and freedom. They lived in rich hunting and foraging grounds, they had lots of free time each day, their levels of chronic stress were incredibly low and they lived in egalitarian societies.

Don't be too quick to envy them, though; they experienced incredible daily challenges, too. A broken leg could mean death and hunting big game like buffalo, bison or woolly mammoths was a dangerous thing, so this was not an easy life on those terms. We've solved some of these problems, though, and through technology we now have the safety net they never had, but in achieving this we have traded our vitality for that privilege. We do have sufficiently advanced technology to swing the pendulum the other way and have the best of both worlds.

What we can do is use the evolutionary lens to look at well-being in a new light and ask new questions. The evolutionary lens is only the starting point and we can use science to guide our way from there.

You are not going to arrive at one prescribed diet, one rigid dogma in this book. Given the evidence we have this is impossible. What you will get is a template that within it allows for a tremendous amount of variation. As Richard Nikoli, author of *Free The Animal, Beyond the Blog,* is fond of reminding us, wild free humans existed from sea level to 16 000 feet and from the equator to the arctic circle. What he means is that they lived in very different environments with different climates, different foods available to them and different challenges.

With all those differences it is impossible to say with certainty that all humans should eat exactly the same things in exactly the same amounts. Through all of that difference, though, we do find some patterns, some commonalities and it's those that offer us a framework in which to operate.

Heuristics

When we operate in very complex areas with so much uncertainty where the scientific information seems to be contradictory and we can't be specialists in everything then it's useful to develop heuristics or 'rules of thumb' to guide us.

You don't need to be able to debate the biochemical ways gluten affects your intestinal wall with a researcher or the way your hormonal system responds to heavy lifting with a biochemist.

It's useful to you to have effective and reasonably accurate rules for navigating the choices you make every day. These rules that are based on sound principles. Principles don't change while the fine details of scientific discovery are always changing. I'm going to guide you over the rough sea of scientific progress in the smooth sailing boat of heuristics.

How do we apply it?

While it is true that every stressor we unpack is a step in the right direction I don't advise the 'baby steps' approach. In my experience, it takes too long for most people to notice a change and get early wins to keep them engaged. It seems like our psychology demands some good short term results in order for us to buy into the whole process. Some people do manage to stick to the 'baby steps' approach but not most. Put simply, we want it now!

By the same token, try to do too much, too soon and you will be overwhelmed. This is the outcome of most crash diets and exercise programmes. They demand too much change too soon. My experience and research shows that people just don't follow through with this approach. Many of the programmes that use before and after photos should have 'after-after' photos so that you can see what has happened a year later. Again, some people do respond to this approach, but most don't.

Unpacking the backpack is the key, removing stressors and adding nutrients while addressing dysfunction of the nervous system. Go too slowly and you get bored, go too quickly and you get overwhelmed. It seems like we're a little like Goldilocks trying to find out what's just right.

The weakness in your genes

The pornography of temptation

While our genes come with the ability to activate health, there is a genetic kryptonite: it's called pornography. Your genes are weak in the face of the dirtiest, nastiest and most lurid porn you can think of: food porn, marketing porn, violence porn, drama porn, sexual porn and health and fitness porn.

Your physiology rewards you for doing things that feed your genes. Your genes expect you to move everyday so when you do, you feel good. Your genes expect you to experience certain tastes so when you do, you feel good. This good feeling comes because these actions activate the reward pathway in your brain. Part of that is the release of the chemical dopamine. Think of it as the reward chemical: go for a run, here's your dopamine; lift some weights, here's your dopamine; eat sweet food, here's your dopamine; practice gratitude, here's your dopamine. You get a stimulus, like movement, and you get a sense of gratification as your reward.

This reward pathway is an amazingly intelligent way that our ancient biology of mind-body helped our ancestors to stay on track, and it still helps us today. It motivates us to seek more of the things that create growth and repair and experience vitality. Our weakness lies in the fact we have found ways of hijacking that reward pathway and seek instant gratification without any of the foreplay nature intended. This is what porn does.

Supernormal stimulation

A supernormal stimulus, or superstimulus, is an exaggerated version of a stimulus to which there is an existing response tendency, or, any stimulus that elicits a response more strongly than the stimulus for which it evolved.

By popular definition porn focuses on sexual imagery, people doing 'dirty' things related to sex. There is a broader view, one which Frank Forencich talks about in his book *Change Your Body, Change The World*. Forencich defines porn as anything that takes us directly from impulse to gratification, bypassing all the anticipation, romance, subtlety, warm up, nurturing that our biology is wired for. It's abrupt and blatant. He says, "It drops you directly into a fantasy realm and pumps you to exhaustion."

Nikolaas Tinbergen, a Dutch biologist, studied animal behaviour and described the effect of pornography, or supernormal stimuli, when he found out that by exaggerating certain physical traits he could make a Herring Gull chick beg for food from a fake model rather than its own parent. He could make a songbird's parent prefer to feed a fake baby bird with a wider beak than a fledgling songbird. He and his team even found that birds preferred plaster eggs that were larger with more exaggerated markings than their own, even though the fake eggs were so big the birds slid off them repeatedly. Give a greylag goose the choice between its own egg and a volleyball and it will choose the volleyball.

Another research team could make the Julodimorpha beetle attempt to mate a beer bottle using the same principle. You've probably noticed similar types of behaviour happening, for example, when an insect flies directly into a candle flame or fire simply because it is bright. These experiments, however bizarre or harmful – Nobel Prizes notwithstanding – give us a clue of our own behaviour.

Supernormal stimuli take over your natural instincts and distort them unrealistically, diminishing your enjoyment and interest in normal stimuli. Once the beetle has seen a beer bottle it will prefer bottles over real beetles. Once you've had fantasy sex with a porn star from a movie, who wants to go back to real people? Why would you want to eat real food once you've tasted all the sweet, salty, fatty, flavoured, food-like products?

Porn is the exaggeration of something we are biologically wired to seek but for which we don't have an 'off' button. Addiction and addiction-like behaviours are the hijacking and overstimulation of our dopamine reward pathways. When we are faced with porn, whether in the form of traditional pornography, certain tastes, drugs or gambling, we can lose all self control and, just as damaging, our interest in real life. In this way sugar and heroin act in a very similar way. Sugar produces a strong dopamine surge but it was fairly rare to the vast majority of our ancestors, so they wouldn't have had this supernormal stimulus.

150

Frank Forencich reminds us that the baseline for our senses is that of wild, free humans. Our ancestor's sensory stimulation was the experience of the Palaeolithic: subtle colours and textures with a mosaic of grass and semi-wooded areas with patterns of grass swaying in the breeze, leaves rustling overhead, or clouds rolling across the sky. Whether it was snowscapes or beach-side environments, our senses were caressed rather than assaulted. Apart from the hunt or an encounter with a predator, life moved very slowly. This is our baseline.

Compare this to the exaggerated reality we live in today. We have bright colours and flashing lights constantly demanding our attention. Magazines have images of airbrushed people whose smiles and curves have been enhanced to promote what we 'should' look like. Intense tastes in food-like products hijack our evolutionary pathway and create cravings. We have a glut of information on our phones, tablets and computers with loud voices all clamouring for our consumer attention. All this sensory porn over-stimulates our senses, promising and delivering instant gratification without any romance, making us want more and more, all the while luring us further and further from real fulfilment.

A specific type of supernormal stimuli is the food-like substances we are surrounded by. We don't classify these as foods but suffice to say that they are laden with injected tastes, many times the intensity we would have ever encountered in nature. Sweet, salty, fatty Franken-foods that hyper stimulate our senses are called hyperpalatable and they trigger our reward pathways like an addict with a hit of heroin. Our will power is belittled in the face of this biological kryptonite. ●

> *Inspiration exists, but it has to find you working.*
> PABLO PICASSO

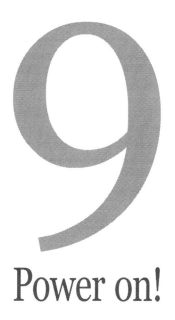

Power on!

A new look at something old.
More than an expensive painkiller.
The human potential movement in practice.
Posture: your new secret weapon?

Chiropractic care

If I gave you a new and fancy food processor and didn't give you the instructions you might only use it to chop up food and that would be useful. But if I then told you a bit more about it, how it could liquidise food to make soups, crush ice to make smoothies and knead mixtures to make bread, then it would be even more useful to you.

When I ask people what they know about Chiropractic they generally tell me one of two things. Either they tell me that they know it's for back pain, neck pain, headaches or sports injuries (which it can be very useful for), or they tell me it's about crunching and cracking bones, (which sounds a little brutal). While Chiropractors are good at relieving many sorts of pain, we are something much more than an elaborate, relatively expensive painkiller.

To find out what it's really about let's look back at what we know. We know that your mind-body is a self-developing, self-regulating ecosystem that is integrated by the nervous system. We know that the health of our whole mind-body relies on the health of each system, and the nervous system is the master coordinator of all the systems. With the nervous system clear we get information from the brain to the body and from the body to the brain. This two-way communication is vital to the optimum function of our mind-body.

How you interact with the outside world is also integrated through your nervous system. Every sunset, piece of music, tasty mouthful of food, every smell and every touch you've ever experienced in your life is processed in your nervous system. To be able to perceive your world and experience the fullness of life you want your nervous system to be crystal clear.

We know that if the structure of our body interferes in any way with our nervous system, either with the messages to or the messages from the brain, then the nervous system dysfunctions. The way this structural interference happens is nuanced, varied and causes lots of confusion. In the end, though, we have a basic set of things that goes wrong. We have a bone that loses its optimal alignment with the rest of the body and we don't have muscles pulling in the direction needed to correct the misalignment. This misalignment can then interfere with the nerve signals either from the brain to the body or from the body to the brain; when this happens it is called a subluxation.

Subluxation creates interference in the signals between the brain and the body and could mean that the cells organs and glands of the body don't get the right information. This would lead to dysfunction and defence mode where they might produce too much or too little of a chemical that, over time it may lead to various forms of disease. Muscles may misfire, deactivate or tighten and our balance and coordination might be affected and lead to injury.

If this subluxation is altering the messages from the body to the brain then it changes how the brain responds to all other information coming into the senses. What research has shown is that misalignment anywhere in the spine disrupts the brain's ability to accurately sense what is going on in the rest of the body. Remember, your nervous system is the conductor of the orchestra that is your mind-body and leads it to play wonderful music in the form of growth and repair chemicals. In cases of subluxation your conductor either can't hear that orchestra properly or can't give them correct direction.

The normal input from the body to the brain is called proprioception and it is a vital nutrient for brain function. It helps to balance the brain and nervous system, specifically the 'fight or flight' and the 'rest and digest' impulses. With a misalignment of the structure of the body we now have a deficiency of proprioception and this is where we see some real problems. Proprioception helps to keep us in growth and repair mode and with it turned down, we begin to move toward defence and decay because, without the full complement of our body to brain signals, we activate the sympathetic (fright or flight) nervous system. The stress pathways and the HPA (hypothalamus-pituitary-adrenal) axis are activated, adding to our stress chemistry.

Proactive beats reactive
When you develop even the smallest amount of dysfunction in the nervous system you will begin to manifest it as defence physiology and it will add to that defence and decay cascade. From a state of defense we get chronic inflammation and all the damage and decay it brings to all parts of your mind-body. It can then silently wreak havoc on your mind-body even though you can't feel it. The reality is that as the dysfunction accumulates it will, together with the other stressors in your system, begin dimming the light of your life, robbing you of your personal performance and human potential.

Even when you are feeling fine, subluxaton could be affecting your health. Because it disturbs the information that your body sends to your brain, your brain can learn to dysfunction. Day by day your mind-body is now forming a new, distorted sense of reality and you might not even know it.

Remember that because stressors will impact different people in different ways and we all have differing amounts of GAP, it's very hard to say what dysfunction might manifest as. For some it might be pain or muscle tension, for others it might be digestive or hormonal disorders and for others it might be memory, mood or learning issues. For this reason I prefer to say that while Chiropractic is effective for many sorts of health challenges it is not a treatment for any specific condition. Rather, Chiropractic is about restoring normal alignment to the structure of the body, to free up nerve signals between brain and body and body and brain and allow us to move from defence to growth, from decay to repair. Chiropractic is more about the brain than it is about the pain.

Internationally Chiropractic is well recognised as safe, natural and effective. It is a non-drug, non-surgical approach to health that is trusted by millions of families everyday.

Adaptability
An effective measure of the balance between growth and defence we currently have is called Heart Rate Variability or HRV. HRV measures how active your 'fight or flight' response is in relation to your 'rest and digest' response. Your 'fight or flight' messages are carried by your sympathetic nervous system and the 'rest and digest', messages are carried in your parasympathetic nervous system.

If you had a heart rate of 60 beats per minute your heart would not beat each second on the second like a metronome. Instead some beats would be closer together and some would be further apart. This variability in the heart beat is HRV. The more variability your heart beats shows, the more balanced your sympathetic and parasympathetic nervous systems are, the better your health, adaptability and resilience.

Poor HRV scores are linked to depression, diabetes, pre-term infants, heart failure, and heart attacks to name but a few. The great news is that research shows that Chiropractic care can improve your HRV.

Other studies directly measured changes in the brain immediately after a Chiropractic correction, called an adjustment, and found that the sympathetic tone of the nervous system was inhibited. This means that Chiropractic can help to move the body from defence and decay into growth and repair.

Yet another research group showed that Chiropractic adjustments improve the adaptability, or neuroplasticity, of the brain as well as inhibit the sympathetic nervous tone.

So not only do we move out of defence but we also a move into growth. Neuroplasticity is important for learning and for helping the brain stay young. We discovered earlier that it plays a central role in your ability to create new habits and truly transform. Adaptability is important for managing stress and solving problems. Just imagine the implications for you and your family if your ability to grow, learn, develop and dance in the chaos of life were enhanced!

You don't have to be in pain to benefit from Chiropractic care!

Blood pressure
Blood pressure is a reliable marker for health; the better it is the more healthy you are. In two separate studies, each looking at different areas of the spine, it has been shown that Chiropractic care improved blood pressure better than placebo. One study found that Chiropractic care was as effective as two blood pressure drugs given in combination.

General health
Numerous studies from around the world have shown that Chiropractic care for subluxations can help you to be healthier in a variety of ways. A 7 year study found that, compared to those who don't, people who see a chiropractor regularly had 60% less hospital admissions and saved on pharmaceutical costs by 85%.

Pregnancy and labour
Using Chiropractic care during pregnancy is a smart move. We love looking after pregnant mums in our practice and they love the results of having Chiropractic checks. Pregnant women who see Chiropractors find they feel less pain and carry more comfortably. Research shows that they also have decreased labour times and need half the pain medications during labour.

Having the structure of your body well-aligned reduces the chances of the use of forceps during birth and the chances of needing an emergency caesarean section.

Some Chiropractic techniques have been shown to be useful to help the baby to turn when it is in the breach position.

Babies, kids and adolescents

My wife and I were fortunate to have very smooth and gentle home delivery with my daughter and she had her first Chiropractic check and adjustment when she was 20 minutes old. Even when everything went so well there were still signs of subluxation in her spine and nervous system. Because it was found early in her life we were able to correct it very easily. One of the biggest joys in my life is giving my daughter a regular Chiropractic check and adjustment if it's required.

Sadly subluxations can occur with even normal births and may be more prevalent when interventions like forceps and caesarean section are used. The majority of babies who have subluxation early on in life never have this addressed.

We see a lot of babies and kids in our practice and they love their Chiropractic adjustments. In the USA, Chiropractors are the most common alternative health providers visited by children and adolescents. When we see kids their parents tell us that they suffer from fewer colds and flu, they have fewer allergies and they sleep better. Parents often bring their kids in for feeding problems, colic, ear infections, bed wetting, asthma and learning difficulties and it is a rare case that does not respond well.

During exam season we see the local school kids and university students come in for a few extra checks because they feel they focus, study and perform better under stress when they are well adjusted.

Safety

Chiropractic care is safe when delivered in the hands of a trained professional. It has a long and well documented history of safety. In 1979 the Government of New Zealand convened a special commission to study Chiropractic. After almost 2 years of research and in 377 pages the report states, "The conspicuous lack of evidence that Chiropractors cause harm or allow harm to occur through neglect of medical referral can be taken to mean only one thing: that Chiropractors have on the whole an impressive safety record."

In Australia some annual statistics tell a story:
* 18 000 deaths from medical treatment errors
* 50 000 injuries by medical treatment errors

- 233 300 suspected adverse drug events
- 41 complaints relating to Chiropractic care.

In children there have been no deaths possibly associated with Chiropractic worldwide in over 40 years while between 2008 and 2012 there were at least 2935 deaths from adverse drug reactions in children in the US.

Compared to general practitioners and medical specialists, Chiropractors have very low rates of malpractice insurance. This reflects the safety of the profession.

Posture

Ultimately, it appears that homeostasis and autonomic regulation are intimately connected with posture.
THE AMERICAN JOURNAL OF PAIN MANAGEMENT

Posture is a very good way to assess the state of your spine and nervous system, but there is a major misunderstanding that needs to be cleared up first. Posture is not how *you* hold your *body* up with muscular effort. Posture is how your *body* holds *you* up when you let yourself breathe out and slump, because your structure holds you up without having to consciously use your muscles. Healthy bodies stay up and back while bodies that are breaking down generally go forward and down.

In a standing position you can breathe in, breathe out and let your body slump. Ideally your shoulders should line up with your ears which should line up with your hips and the middle of your feet *with your muscles relaxed*. If your head, shoulders, hips or whole body sways or slumps forward then that's evidence that your body is structurally misaligned with subluxation and your nervous system is dysfunctioning; you have dis-ease and you are doing defence and decay.

Forward posture decreases the capacity of your heart and lungs by up to 30% and it influences your blood pressure, predisposes you to injury and pain of various sorts and degrades your movement patterns. Forward posture is also linked with decreased energy, moods and a poor mental state.

For people with forward posture over a long time the news is very bad. The more your body stoops forward, the higher your chance of having a heart attack and dying early of many causes.

Since it is a sign of poor health, evolution has made poor posture visually unappealing and good posture very attractive to us. Looking at a body that is upright with shoulders back and eyes looking straight ahead is captivating.

Headspace

The benefits of effortlessly upright posture go way beyond the physical. The link between your mind and your body is evident once again when studies show that people exhibit more confidence with open posture, and that posture affects your cognitive and emotional state. An upright posture is linked to a positive mentality about yourself and your life.

Studies show that when you are sad your head goes forward and your body slumps and the reverse happens when you are happier. This link works both ways, though: when people adopt more upright postures they are more positive about themselves and more confident in their ability to navigate life. When people adopt slumped postures the opposite is true.

While these studies are useful the subjects in them were using their muscles to hold them upright. We've learned that this approach to posture can only give you transient change because it does not solve the underlying cause of forward posture.

By working with the body to structurally correct the subluxations it is possible to have your body hold you up effortlessly instead of straining to hold your body up. Not only could this help you to be more confident and optimistic but it could also help you to be happier with your body and more accepting of yourself.

What about the kids

Kids growing up in this technology heavy era are showing some worrying signs. Having their head down as they are absorbed by a phone, tablet or laptop puts incredible strain on the spine and nervous system. Heavy school bags cause twists in their body structure that adds insult to the injury that is prolonged sitting at home and at school. I've noticed that kids with learning issues and emotional volatility tend to have particularly slumped posture and respond well to correction.

How?

When you get subluxations – structural misalignments that your body does not have muscles pulling in the right direction to self-correct – your structure loses its leverage and begins to slump forward. In addition to causing dysfunction in your nervous system and general state of dis-ease, as you slump forward you put pressure on your organs and impede their function. Subluxations create an imbalance between your sympathetic and parasympathetic nervous system function and puts you further into the 'fight or flight' range: this creates defence and decay.

In addition to robbing your brain of the proprioceptive signals that it uses as stimulation, you also begin to create tension on your brain and spinal cord. The spinal cord is protected by the bones of your spine and is suspended between the brain at top of your neck and the sacrum at the base of your spine. As it relays messages between the brain and body it gives off a tone, or frequency, of these impulses, like a string on a violin. In a normal body there should be some slack in the spinal cord giving it a certain tone but, when the body slumps forward, the tension increases and the tone changes from growth to defence.

The change in tension and tone has an effect on the entire body, physically straining the brain through the brain stem. This mechanical tension can alter the messages going between brain and body and it can lead to changes in blood flow and chemical imbalances in the delicate neural tissue.

The spinal cord is tensioned when a body slumps forward in breakdown when you have subluxation, and your mind-body is forced to go into defence and decay when this happens. There is one last step that makes this a tougher problem to solve than most people think. We already know that this isn't a case of just sitting up straight, because you have no muscles pulling in the direction needed to correct the subluxation. This is one of the things your body cannot self correct.

The secondary problem is the plastic bag like substance that surrounds the spinal cord and brain, called the meninges, can get stuck. This meningeal 'sleeve' can get twisted and distorted with subluxation and can form adhesions that further affect the tension on the spinal cord and can fix the subluxations in place.

Complete structural correction

Through many years of study around the world and many courses and seminars, as well as working with people's bodies for over 15 years, I've found a way of working with people that is different to most other forms of bodywork. Most Chiropractors, physiotherapists, osteopaths and massage therapists place people face down on a bed to do their work and push from the back of the body to the front. This approach does result in profound improvements in health and also pain relief for people a lot of the time.

A revolutionary approach to working with bodies suggests that working with bodies the other way around might be an even better idea. Your body has muscles that can pull on the spine going forward and side to side but because the spine is the furthest backward point of the body you have no muscles pulling directly backwards. This basic fact suggests that bones stuck forward are stuck in a direction the body cannot self correct, while bones stuck in other directions are self correctable.

Bones stuck forward then lose their leverage and the body begins to slump forward. By correcting only these subluxations and allowing the body to correct the misalignments that it can self correct we can work with the body in a far more powerful way.

Advanced Biostructural Correction™ (ABC™) is the revolutionary method of body work that does just that. ABC™ consistently creates change in people's bodies and produces results that other people just talk about. In the book *Straight Forward: Why Forward Posture Affects Your Health and How To Fix It*, Dr Hooman Zahedi says that ABC™ is different because:
- It's a protocol with a predictable outcome
- It allows the body to unwind through previous injuries
- Allows the body to get back to an effortlessly upright, more resilient position
- It focuses on correcting only what the body cannot and allowing the body to unwind through those misalignments that it can.

While there is lots of validity to what other Chiropractors do when they correct what the body cannot self-correct, ABC™ is the only method of bodywork that I practice and that my family and I have done on us. ●

10

Be the balance

What colour is your lens?
Be here now.
Network for well-being.
The game of life.

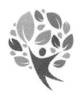

Think!

Every thought and feeling that you have in your mind has an immediate and measurable effect on your body through your nervous system. Your muscles tighten and relax according to your state of mind. Your heart beat changes according to your state of mind. Your organs and glands change their function according to your state of mind. Chemicals called neuropeptides flood your body, communicating every thought or emotion you are experiencing at every moment, everyday to every cell in your body, influencing their activity.

There are whole fields of research that are studying how the mind affects the immune system (psychoneuroimmunology), your hormones (psychoneuroendocrinology), your digestive system (psychoneurogastroenterology) and how it affects the structure of your body. The days of doctors claiming that the problem is 'in your head' to explain away things they did not understand is now long gone. Your mind, your thoughts and your emotions are having a direct impact on your health.

Headspace rocks

Have you ever thought about your state of mind as a nutrient? Have you even considered your state of mind a stressor?

It's easy to understand that to a wild, free human, a threat such as a lion would set off the stress response. Living in Africa I've been face to face with a lion, thankfully with iron bars and a few metres between us, and I can tell you that the primal response in my body was powerful. His low, menacing growl resonated in my solar plexus and my primal brain was telling me that I didn't need to be there. If you've never come up close to a lion then an equivalent might be a masked gunman in your home.

Your brain, through your senses, perceives the threat and then relays that information to the sympathetic nervous system and the HPA axis, which then sets off the stress response. In the stress response your mind-body suppresses functions not needed for immediate survival: digestion, immune system, reproduction and growth are all shut down, you don't need them if you're facing a masked gunman.

Acute mental and emotional stressors like a lion would last just minutes at a time and if you survived, then your physiological stress response would fade away within a few hours. The problem is that although you and I inherited this ancient biology, we don't live in that world anymore. We have a near constant stream of signals to our brain that can be perceived as stressors if we let them. An impending deadline at work, a test at school, a mother in law coming to stay, trouble with your spouse, kids or best friend, or a pile of unpaid bills are all lower grade stressors that your mind-body reacts to over a much longer time, and they accumulate.

We can even imagine stressors that don't actually exist anymore. We can remember past stressors and feel the effect they have on us. Post traumatic stress disorder (PTSD) is an extreme example of a stressor, where victims of trauma will relive the event over and over again and each time the stress response will ravage their mind-body. You don't have to have PTSD to experience this effect: every time you replay an argument, a confrontation, a breakup or a loss, your mind-body is reliving the stress response.

We can even project a stressor into the future by imagining a confrontation, a deadline or a test and your mind-body begins to live in that future event through the effect your nervous system and the chemical cascades you produce.

The accumulation of every mental and emotional stressor in your life, both real and imagined is an indelible scar in your mind-body. As Mark Twain said, "I am an old man and have known a great many troubles but most of them never happened."

Perception is everything

Imagine there is a computer malfunction which results in a freak accident when a traffic light indicates green for two directions of traffic at the same time. Two cars end up colliding in the middle of the intersection. One driver gets out of his car, angrily shouting and cursing.

"Why does it always happen to me? The dog next door kept me up all last night; I stubbed my toe this morning; because the geyser is broken I had a cold shower and a fight with my wife about the plumber; I'm late for work and now, to top it all, this happens!"

The other driver gets out of his car and says, "Wow, we're lucky to be alive."

The same thing happens for both men, a crash where neither was to blame, yet their reactions are so vastly different. Their perception of the incident is completely divergent that it seems like two separate accidents.

There is a lens through which we each view the world, a lens that made one man shout and curse while it caused the other to simply feel grateful. My lens makes me see certain things in a shopping centre while my wife sees very different things in the same space. Each of us has a unique lens and because of this we filter events through that lens with completely different experiences.

A friend of mine was sharing his frustration about his unreasonable boss. She had shouted at him and his team for the delay in delivering a project. When we sat down over a cup of tea and I asked whether the rest of his team felt the same, he said that they didn't. Apparently some of his team felt that their boss was completely reasonable in her anger because they had dropped the ball; they felt excited to work even harder and produce something special. They had been on the same project under the same boss and were in the same meeting, yet they had a different perception of the boss. They had a different lens through which they perceived and experienced the event.

What one person sees as stressful and damaging might reveal significance and growth to someone else; it's a nutrient for their mind-body. A lens that colours our view of life determines whether an event is a stressor or a nutrient.

The lens through which we see the world is our philosophy of life, our values and beliefs. It's mostly subconscious and it directs where and what our conscious mind perceives at every moment of everyday. The driver who believed the world was out to get him today could have found it impossible to see how the second driver could feel gratitude for the crash. My friend found it impossible to see how his boss was being reasonable.

How you perceive the world and what you give significance to has profound effects on your physiology and can influence activation or deactivation of your genes. In 2008 researchers studied gene expression in youngsters with asthma between 9 and 18 years old. They showed them videos of awkward or ambiguous situations and asked them how threatening they found them. Those who found the videos more threatening showed a big change in their gene-expression scores while those who saw less threat showed very little change.

Your thoughts and feelings flip genetic switches and produce physiological changes throughout your mind-body. In the study they assessed the genes that affected the stress response which leads to defence and decay. The bigger the threat perceived, the more their mind-body was seeking defence and decay.

166

Most of our values and beliefs are subconsciously downloaded while we are young. Through our mothers, fathers, teachers and preachers we form our lens by the age of 6 and it directs our experience of life from then on. Whether we are smart or not, whether we are good enough or not, whether money is good or bad, whether we have conservative or liberal views of the world – these are usually engrained in us by the tender age of 6.

If you have not clearly defined what your values and beliefs are, if you have allowed your map and compass to be passively downloaded and reinforced through life, then you are running through life half blind. You'll be like the driver that thought the world was out to get him or my friend who thought his boss was being unreasonable.

Presence

Thankfully there is a way to make this subconscious programming more conscious; there is a way to become aware of your philosophy of life, your values and beliefs, and to wake up to them.

When I lived in Scotland I used to take two busses to and from work each day. Now, winter in Scotland is cold and wet. The sun rises at about 9:30 and goes down at around 16:00 and that year we didn't see the sun very much, we had 40 days and 40 nights of continuous rain. The newspapers called it 'biblical rain'. Waiting at bus stops at 5:30 to get to work and to leave work at 19:30 was not fun and you can bet that I grumbled under my breath most days as I waited.

On my route we often had a man who was, to put it nicely, not a functional member of society. He was clearly disturbed in some way. He rode the busses all day, every day, going nowhere. If he was on your bus you tried not to engage him because, when he wasn't talking to himself quietly or ranting and raving about something indecipherable, he would look straight at you and then start talking to you as if you were a friend or a family member. He would talk about things that had happened in the past and things that would happen in the future. He was always talking, either to himself or at you. What you had to say in return or whether you said anything didn't seem to matter to him at all.

At one point I saw him walk past empty seats on the bus and then proceed to stand in the aisle complaining that there were no empty seats available. I heard him complain that the bus driver was driving too fast when we were standing still at a bus stop. He had departed from reality in a number of ways and was clearly insane. You could liken his behaviour to being unconscious because he was not aware of reality and was in a dream-like delusion.

On one such trip I was listening to a recording of Ekhart Tolle, an author and teacher on the subject of our minds and consciousness, and watching the man. Tolle made a startling observation that struck me so deeply in that moment that it changed my perception of reality altogether. He said that when we are engaging in conversation in our own head, when we are carried away by our 'mind chatter' we are just as insane as the man I was watching: we are just as unconscious, we are just as delusional.

I'd missed my stop on the bus a few times because I was lost in some pattern of thought; as a doctor I had sometimes missed what people had said to me because there was a conversation in my head about their symptoms or even their hair style or their clothes; sometimes I find myself still mulling over what someone said to me hours before; as husband and father I have looked right at my wife or daughter and not been aware of what they were saying because I was carried away by my internal dialogue.

What I realised then was what people have been teaching for years; *you are not your mind*. Your mind is a useful tool for navigating the world but *you are not your mind*. If you don't know this or you're too wrapped up by the constant stream of stuff your mind thinks then you are not fully conscious of reality. You are not fully present in any given moment and you are missing out on the most amazing gift.

Your internal dialogue gives you the gift of finding out what your philosophy of life is. The thoughts and feelings that constantly come and go as part of the mind's meandering ebb and flow are all results of our core values and beliefs, and by becoming aware of that flow we can locate the source.

It's called the present for a reason

Love, certainty, gratitude and presence are our default state of being, they represent mental vitality. They are our innate state of mind and when we depart from that state we are toxic and deficient in our mental and emotional habits. What that really means is that joy and fulfilment are our natural states of being: they are within us all the time. Our ability to cut through the detritus that daily life serves us and focus on what matters is all that stands between us and happiness.

168

Does that sound too good to be true? Does it sound too easy? It is neither. Through my work with thousands of people I have seen lives transformed in an instant when this realisation hits. But it's only the beginning. After the realisation that mental vitality really is inside all the time comes the practice of stripping through the layers of stressors that daily life throws at us, plus the layers or stressors we've accumulated in the past. It's like realising that you have the ability to be the best sprinter in the world, all you have to do is train hard day in and day out to get there.

At any given moment of any given day your capacity to be aware and to truly experience life is determined by your level of awareness in that moment. What some have called mindfulness or Present Time Consciousness (PTC) is the thing that determines the quality of your experience of life.

Our ability to be present is a key factor in the search for happiness. Mental vitality is like a clear, sunny sky over our heads: it's always there while our thoughts, feelings and moods are like clouds. From the ground, the clouds may temporarily cover the sunshine but above the clouds the sunshine is always there.

The challenge is when we continuously identify with and are subject to that meandering flow that is our mind. When we are in that state we are under the clouds and believe the sun is gone. When we are under the clouds we will live in the future or the past as we relive old events, or imagine new events over and over and over. Each time we think about stressful events our mind-body re-lives them as if they have just happened. The simulations you run in your mind affect your body directly and instantaneously create mind-body states of either growth or defence.

When you become aware of this fact and begin to practise mindfulness, you become more aware that you have indeed begun a process of awakening from a subconscious dream-state of insanity that is the mind.

Your thoughts are like the incessant flow of traffic on a motorway. Each thought in your mind is like one of those cars, hurtling down the highway. When you are mind-identified then you sit in each 'car', having the thought until the next one takes you, switching as each new thing grabs your attention. If you've ever used the internet, clicking through links taking you in so many different directions with so many tabs open that your computer slows down or crashes, then you've had this experience.

What most of us think should happen when we meditate or practice mindfulness is that we clear our mind, that we should jump out onto our thought highway and stop all the 'cars'. Well, the physics of that situation is exactly what plays out in our minds: we get run over by the flow of thoughts and feelings and end up giving up.

In reality the practise of mindfulness through meditation in all its forms helps us to learn to sit next to the highway of our thoughts and observe the flow. In the beginning we might be able to observe for a little while and then get carried away by one or more of the thoughts that go whizzing by before remembering to return to the place of observation. The goal is not to stop the 'cars'. The goal is simply to observe your thoughts with curiosity and compassion and without judgement.

You don't have to be a vegetarian or sit cross-legged on a mat chanting in order to meditate. Classic meditation is one set of techniques but there are many others. Any form of movement where you are focused on your body and its actions can be meditative. Qui Gong, Tai Chi and yoga are classic eastern practises of using the body to observe the mind. Yoga is not a practise for becoming more flexible (that is an allopathic thought), it is a spiritual practice using the body to prepare the mind for contemplation.

You can reshape almost any movement into mindfulness. Running or walking where you maintain internal awareness by focusing on your breath. Your footfall or your technique can be meditative. The same goes for lifting weights, cycling, swimming, rowing, skipping or any other physical activity. So long as you maintain a strong awareness either of your body and its motion, your breath, or of the sights and sounds of your external surrounds, you will help focus your mind and become meditative.

The art of mindfulness can be carried into any activity you do on any day. When you're cooking, turn off the TV, turn off the iPod and do each thing, one at a time. Washing, chopping and peeling vegetables where you maintain single focus on the task at hand is mindfulness. Frying food in a pan and concentrating on just that frying food in the pan is mindfulness. While I'm typing this I'm focussing on the sounds of my fingers on the keyboard and the stream of thoughts flowing through my fingertips. Each time my mind wonders I notice it and simply refocus on the sound of my fingers on the keyboard. Some days it's easy, some days it's not. Each day is different and each day is practise.

Significance

D r Herbert Benson, founder of the Harvard Mind-Body Institute says it best: "Neurological research reveals that before we consciously colour the world around us with our thinking and acquired beliefs, brain mechanisms mark our perceptions, forming opinions and assigning emotional values. Before we even have a chance to mull over the presence of a new sight or sound, regions of our brain react by assigning an initial but influential value to it. These automatic attitudes make us incapable of utter objectivity or neutrality, in more profound ways than we've ever suspected."

Benson is saying that an event happens around us and we observe it as it comes in through our external senses. As soon as that stimulus reaches our brain, we automatically and subconsciously evaluate what that stimulus means. There is no time where we are consciously evaluating that new event without our pre-programmed values and beliefs. As soon as we are consciously aware of something our subconscious values and beliefs have already assigned a level of importance to the input. Stimuli of high importance are given preference over stimuli of low importance.

Your values and beliefs – your philosophy of life – is the lens through which your subconscious perceives and processes events instantly. Your lens creates a hierarchy of values that determine how you see the world.

The lens
Things that are highest in your hierarchy of values will get the most significance because they matter more to you, and you will we have more time, more money and more energy for them. You will be most disciplined and organised around your higher values. Things that are lower down, that are of less significance, matter less and your perception becomes that you don't have time, energy and money for these things. You will be least disciplined and organised around these lower values.

Dr John Demartini, a human behavioural specialist, had a client who wanted him to work with his 12 year old son. While his son was a bright youngster, he was doing poorly at school and he spent all his time playing computer games. The father really wanted his son to do well, so Dr Demartini spoke to the boy and found he placed a high value on computer games. Now because he placed a high value on it, he could play for hours; he could make time when there was no time to do it. He would save his money and concentrate all his resources so that he could get the latest games and updates. He could concentrate his mind effortlessly while playing and understanding the games and he could remember the different stages of the games very quickly and with surprising ease.

The same boy placed a very low value on his schoolwork, specifically history, and he struggled to find time and focus for his homework. He didn't have the energy or concentration and would forget what he'd read straight away. Dr Demartini asked the boy how he made time and where he got the motivation and found the focus for playing the games, but the boy couldn't really tell him exactly, other than how much he loved doing it.

When asked why the boy lacked the time, attention and the motivation for his homework, all the boy did was come up with a list of excuses, like having too much homework or having sports practise; or his teachers giving him the wrong things; or things that were too hard for him; or his parents being on his back; or his siblings being the issue. He was very much a victim when he spoke about these things.

> *Your actions scream so loudly at people*
> *that they cannot hear what you are saying.*
> ANON

Dr John Demartini best teaches this value hierarchy and its effect on our lives and he is famous for saying that, "Your life demonstrates your values." What he means is that if you look at where you have been most disciplined, resourceful, organised and energised you will find your high values: what you find most significant. If you look at where you are least organised, resourceful, disciplined and energetic you will find your lowest values.

When we make excuses for not doing something, we're usually justifying the fact that it's low down on our hierarchy of values.

If we're having trouble consistently doing the things we need to do to experience good health and have energy and focus and attention, but we can come up with a whole list of excuses, then we can assume that health and well-being are lower down on our list of values. This would explain why some of the things you might have tried to do in the past to get healthy seemed to peter off or be short-term, because other things in life got in the way. I'm not moralising here, rather suggesting a reason why you are where you are and how you might want to change to be able to move forward.

Lead your life of significance

When you align your life with your values, when you are clear with what your values are and you take action every day to realise those values, then you will lead a life of significance in a way that matters to you. You don't have to be a sports star, a saint, a world leader or a business mogul to lead a life of significance, but you do have to lead a life of congruence in a way that matters to *you*.

CASE HISTORY 6:
Beating fatigue

JODI CAME TO ME a few years ago with chronically low energy to the point where she could only budget 4 hours of useful time a day before she would feel exhausted. She couldn't spend much quality time with her kids and could not even hold down a part time job, where once she had been a highly regarded consultant. She couldn't be the mother, wife, lover and consultant she wanted to be. Getting out of bed was a chore, climbing stairs took her ages and she could hardly hold herself upright in the afternoon.

She came to me with one condition: she didn't think it was a psychological problem and didn't want to do any headspace work. I reluctantly agreed and we started our journey together.

After her initial phase of Chiropractic care she had energy for at least 8 hours of productive time on most days. This was a great improvement in a short amount of time. Jodi was more alert, more mobile and a happier person. Then we worked on her nutrition. We got her moving more and worked on her sleeping patterns and she improved some more, reaching up to 10 hours of good, quality time every day. But then we hit a ceiling. We modified her energy intake, her movement and her sleep but nothing seemed to make a difference; come 4pm everyday she was so fatigued she had to go to bed.

I recommended that we try some headspace work, but she resisted. I believed that this was the missing piece of the puzzle. Jodi resisted to the point that she stopped coming to see me and I didn't hear from her for some months.

Then she called and said she was ready to have a 'powerful conversation': that's the term I use for a meaningful exploration of our inner most lives, that part we usually keep hidden away from everyone. Jodi and I sat down and did a values exercise that gave us a good idea of what her highest values are. After about an hour Jodi had tears in her eyes and we had a clear list in front of us. Jodi assumed that her family was her highest priority so she put their welfare above everything else in her life, including her own health and career.

When she realised that her highest value was her career, that this was where she was most inspired, creative and resourceful, she broke down into more tears. She felt torn between being a good mother and a great professional. This on-going internal conflict where she was feeling torn every minute of every hour was sapping her energy and contributing to her fatigue. We explored what being a good mum meant to her and she spoke about giving her children all of her time and energy, but when I asked her to look back on what had happened when she had tried to do that it was almost too much for her.

We decided to experiment: Jodi was going to find out if being a happy woman who was fulfilled by her career would also help her to be a better mum. She started doing small consulting roles with the energy she had, which did take her away from her family sometimes.

The more she did the consulting work, the better she felt. In just a few weeks Jodi was back to operating through a full day, being able to work 4 days a week and then spend 3 full days with her kids.

The last time I spoke to Jodi she was completing her MBA and was taking 3 months off to travel with her family. Her children were happy that they had they mum back and she was happy she had her life back and her sex life had never been better, too!

Jodi is just one example of how someone has realigned their lives and felt a massive increase in energy to experience vitality. Sometimes the shift is big like a change in job, country or life partner and sometimes it's a small change like starting to read different books. One thing is for certain, though; if you have a mismatch between your values and your life then your well-being will suffer and you will live a life of regrets.

Incongruence leads to destruction

If you are living a life that does not align with your highest values, if you've let society dictate what you should or should not do then you will experience defence and decay. Internally, your mind-body will exhibit the incongruence that we are creating externally and we will sacrifice our personal performance and human potential.

Your bigger life is one where you act everyday in accordance with your own values. Whether that be in your family, your career, your sport, your service to humanity, your faith or anything else you hold as most significant to you. Finding out your values and beliefs, your philosophy of life, all starts by cultivating mindfulness and presence so that you can hear the ramblings of your mind and realise that you are not your mind.

> *Your experiences today will influence the molecular composition of your body for the next two to three months or, perhaps, for the rest of your life. Plan your day accordingly.*
> STEVE COLE, UCLA

Discover your higher values, visit http://thrivelifestyle.solutions/why

What's your greatest asset?

Once you have an idea of your highest values, you can begin to use the inspiration, organisation, resourcefulness and dedication to those high values to live a fulfilled life.

Whether its family, money, travel or your work which is most important to you, you can't really fulfil these values or enjoy the fruits of your labour if your mind-body is not functioning well. By aligning well-being and your highest values you can find higher levels of personal performance and unlock your human potential.

Living life at 8-10/10 is the only way for you to really fulfil those high values and to lead the bigger life you're looking for. Without vitality, you'll feel like Jodi: budgeting your energy every day and feeling torn, frustrated and confused. Imagine knowing what your purpose in life is. Imagine clearly feeling your true calling and then not being able to show up and fulfil that purpose because your mind-body was stuck in defence and decay? How frustrating would that feel? How much regret would course through your mind-body every day, knowing you'd squandered your life on the altar of mediocrity?

If you are clear on your life's purpose, then making sure your brain and body are integrated, that your spine is aligned and that your nervous system is primed with Chiropractic care becomes a necessity and not a luxury.

If you can truly realise how vitality will help you fulfil your highest values then you'll begin to find that eating real food becomes easier and the junk that used to tempt you no longer has a hold on you.

If you know that vitality helps you achieve your most meaningful goals then movement every day becomes a pleasure and excuses will dissolve.

If you unmistakably connect vitality to your great purpose then energy levels soar. You'll be inspired to take action on your purpose and embrace both pleasure and pain in pursuit of it. Instead of being side tracked by the many distractions that make the world seem chaotic you'll begin to dance through the chaos with grace, lightness and ease.

Connection

> *Day by day, week by week, your genes are in a conversation*
> *with your surroundings. Your neighbours, your family, your feelings*
> *of loneliness: they don't just get under your skin,*
> *they get into the control rooms of your cells.*
> DAVID DOBBS, THE SOCIAL LIFE OF GENES

Isolation *vs* Intimacy?
We are social creatures and we thrive being connected to people who matter to us. As wild free humans we would have existed with 30-150 people with whom we

shared very strong links. We would have gone out to find food together; we would have cooked and eaten it together. We would have helped to raise their kids and they would have helped to raise ours. We would have celebrated and we would have commiserated together. Their survival and our survival would have been intertwined. Those that had stronger social bonds than the rest of the group would have had a better chance of surviving than an outsider would have.

Contrast that with your ever expanding list of connections, your 'network' and your Facebook friends, and think about how many of them you are actually connected to. How many of their secrets do we know and hold non-judgementally? How many of them do we love despite knowing their flaws?

The feeling of isolation is a potent risk factor for ill health and early death and is the equivalent of smoking 15 cigarettes a day or having high blood pressure. It is twice as deadly as obesity. Loneliness weakens your immune system and puts you at risk of high blood pressure, heart attack and strokes. A lack of social ties is strongly associated with mental decline, poor physical conditioning and poor balance and co-ordination.

> *Social isolation is the best-established, most robust social or psychological risk factor for disease out there. Nothing can compete.*
> STEVE COLE PHD

Loneliness is a silent plague that we once thought was reserved for the elderly, but we're beginning to realise that it's hurting young people the most. In 2010 the Mental Health Foundation in the United Kingdom found loneliness to be a bigger problem in 18-34 year olds than it was for the over 55's. Amongst our technological expansion of acquaintances we are sorely lacking real connection.

Digital correspondence, whether that be email, text, audio or video, lacks the full range of inputs your primal mind-body craves. We've evolved as social creatures and we expect a wide variety of communication to help us bond with people. Tone, pitch and tempo of voice, full body language, facial expression, scent, eye contact, touch, physical appearance, blink rate and many other non-verbal cues are transmitted with in-person communication to the point that our brain waves, breathing and heart rate become synchronous after a few moments of interacting. This is true connection.

In an SMS you don't get the tone of voice or body language of the person; you don't see their facial expression. Even a video chat doesn't tell you how the person is breathing, how their body moves or how they smell. In the age of digital communication where we are all staring at screens we get precious little intimacy, in fact we get a deficiency of connection. As my wife says, "There is no sarcasm font!."

We can confidently say that a deficiency of social connection leads to a state of defence and decay. From studies in bees and birds to monkeys and humans, research suggests that what happens in our social circle affects the expression of our genes in very strong ways.

Greg Wray, an evolutionary biologist at Duke University who has focused on gene expression for over a decade says, "You suddenly realise birds are hearing a song and having massive, widespread changes in gene expression in just 15 minutes. Something big is going on."

In the animal world, what happens in their social life affects the expression of their genes and it affects you and I just as much.

Survival benefits
Knowing that you are connected to and supported by your band – your tribe – confers and activates growth and repair pathways in your mind-body.

Gay men with HIV live longer healthier lives if they are openly gay rather than closeted. Gay men without HIV who were closeted suffer from cancer and infectious diseases at higher rates than openly gay men.

In a study of 103 healthy women, those who were stressed showed changed gene activity up to 6 months later and the change in gene expression was defence and decay.

Yale psychologist Joan Kaufman found that children with social support (defined as at least monthly contact with a trusted adult figure) were protected from long term effects of severe abuse. Or to look at it another way, the lack of support made them more susceptible to the effects of severe abuse.

In all these studies, what is clear again and again is that our ancient biology expects connection to others. It is a nutrient. Isolation is a deficiency of a genetically required

178

nutrient and has effects on our well-being from the genetic level triggering defence and decay throughout our mind-body.

Connection to people who support our values and dreams is essential. Being surrounded by people who do not align with your values and dreams is toxic. Take steps to find and forge relationships with people who share your outlook on life and are willing to challenge and support you on your way to greatness.

Connection to earth

We've explored how we are ecosystems living as animals within a wider ecosystem and the genes inside our cells need a certain stimulus to activate them into growth and repair. Through our long history we have been living in deep connection and communication with nature. Only in the last few metaphorical seconds of our existence have we separated ourselves from the earth and domesticated ourselves inside our human zoo. Our genes continue to expect connection with nature in various forms and if we aren't making that connection then we're experiencing a deficiency that leads us to defence and decay.

In some startling studies from Japan participants walked in or viewed a forest setting for less than 10 minutes. This unleashed a whole cascade of cellular, hormonal and chemical changes. Cortisol, one of the major chemicals of the chronic stress response dropped; heart rate, blood pressure and the fight or flight activity of the nervous system balanced to growth and repair levels; levels of immune cells called Natural Killer or NK cells that fight off infections and are strongly anti-cancer went up!

Your brain and nervous system is an information gathering miracle. Every sight, sound, smell, taste and touch in your environment is gathered and absorbed every second of every day. Thankfully we're not consciously aware of this constant information tsunami because our brains are very good at filtering most of the noise before it reaches our conscious awareness, but they all have an effect on our physiology. Some estimates say that we are only aware of 50 bits of information every second, while our brain receives more than 3 000 000 000 000 bits from inside and outside our body!

What this means is that despite our best efforts to focus our attention on what matters to us we will absorb every news report and advert on the radio; every car hooter, bumper sticker, flashing sign, billboard and flyer on our way to work or school. Every flashing alert on your phone, tablet or computer, every email, every advert on the net and every word the people around you say is absorbed, even if you aren't aware of it.

Contrast this to the gentle pattern of grass swaying in the wind or the sound of leaves rustling in the trees. Think of the sound of wind and waves on a beach or the feeling of tree bark under your hands. These are the softer, easier, more natural signals that your nervous system is hardwired to expect. These signals are nutrients and produce growth and repair responses while the urban milieu is a toxin and promotes defence and decay.

Knowing this, it makes sense that the 'forest bathing' group experienced such amazing changes, particularly with their immune system. What it shows us once more is how a seemingly small change, such as going for a walk in a forest, can produce a massive change. Take it a step further and go camping for 3 days and the effect is much more pronounced. Now add this to a lifestyle where you are eating and moving in biologically appropriate ways and you will have an avalanche of growth and repair, leading you to open new doors of vitality so that you can lead your bigger life.

Enrich your senses

There are two key ways to get your nature fix and the first is the most powerful. Get outside as often as you can. Whether that's a small walled off garden or a few days in the bush, get outside. Take your meditations, your workouts and your meetings outside and enjoy the boost in focus, productivity, performance and creativity that being outside gives you. While you're out there take a few moments each day to notice the patterns of nature. Enjoy the feeling of grass or the bark of a tree, the smell of flowers or rain, the visual pattern of branches in a tree and the sound of the wind rustling the leaves. Each of these sights and sounds has the power to reactivate your mind-body's ability to grow and repair and lead you to vitality.

For those times when you're outside, go barefoot. Apart from strengthening your feet and legs and improving your posture and balance, it relieves many forms of pain and helps prevent injury. You'll feel more connected to planet earth. Get grass, sand and dirt between your toes. It may take a while to get comfortable with the increased amount of information your feet are receiving and it's an amazing way to get more connected with your body and nature.

180

If getting outside isn't your thing, or you find it hard to accommodate it in your lifestyle, then bring nature inside. Bring some indoor plants into your space and place pictures of natural scenes on your walls or ceilings. We've looked at what a picture can do but plants provide a similar effect while also detoxifying the air you breathe.

You are a reflection of the environment you live in

As we're addressing our own health and we realise that we are part of a greater whole we must consider the health of our planet. This is not a treatise on the devastation we are wreaking on our home planet; I don't expect that information would be new to you. What you might need to know, however, is how this affects you directly.

On a practical level, knowing where your food comes from and how it was produced is the ideal way to become more aware of your environment. Wild, free humans would know exactly where their food came from because they would have had to hunt and gather it for themselves.

Do you eat fresh fruit and vegetables farmed locally or are they chemically treated, frozen and shipped to you from afar? Is your plant matter irradiated? What farming practises are used to produce the fresh produce you eat? Is it sustainably produced or genetically modified? Were the animals treated well or with cruelty?

It is impossible for you to be at the highest levels of vitality and live in a sick environment; you are an ecosystem within an ecosystem.

Gratitude

Gratitude is one of our default states of being. In my experience, gratitude is a doorway to profound growth and repair and is an essential requirement for a life of vitality. Expressing gratitude can help you to transform your life. It can raise your level of mental and emotional function and help you to make better decisions.

If you're living a life of chronic stressors that drain your mental and emotional energy it's often hard to make qualified decisions about nutrition and movement because those superstimuli, like processed food-like substances and lazing on the couch, seem like the path of least resistance. A state of gratitude helps us to hack the system, dramatically reducing our levels of stress and freeing up the necessary faculties to make better choices.

Life is better when you feel blessed, when you can look around and say thank you for what you have and not focus on what you don't have. It's tempting to think that gratitude comes from having what you want. You see yourself giving thanks if you have money, a loving family, maybe a house on the beach, but there are ungrateful, unhappy people with all of these things and there are poor people full of gratitude even though they have very few if any material possessions in life. So, gratitude really comes from your perception.

Gratitude is a cultivated state of mind; like a flower it will blossom when you feed it, but it will wilt if you ignore it. A state of gratitude is very important because of the power you achieve when you are in a state of gratitude. You're going to be challenged in your journey and you're going to want to be able to bear these challenges with grace and ease and lightness so that you can make the best decisions possible under the most challenging circumstances. If you let those old beliefs rule you, then you'll face these challenges in the same way you have always done and nothing will change.

Gratitude helps you unlock deeper vaults of peace and resourcefulness so you can move in new directions. Gratitude is a powerful state of consciousness when your head and your heart are open and you're aligned. If you have limiting beliefs that are holding you back, you'll continue to hit the same old walls and come up with the same old excuses. Gratitude will help you to rise above those old walls, transcend them and go through them. Gratitude arises from how you interpret the world around you – your values and beliefs.

It's the natural feeling that comes from believing that you are fortunate and from truly appreciating the people and things in your life. While it's innate to us, it's also something you can re-learn if you seem to have lost it. To begin we have to stop and become aware of the roses before you can learn how to smell them. You can't have gratitude for something you don't notice. You can make this appreciative approach to roses in life a habit. There's no need to completely ignore and deny the ugliness in the world, but we have to habitually begin to become aware of beautiful things.

You've learned how every thought that you have develops nerve pathways that fire together and wire together in the brain, and thinking in a certain way, repetitively, means that we will reinforce pathways running in the same direction, making it easier to be in that state in the future. This makes it possible to lift your consciousness so you can experience new levels of awareness and gratitude and new possibilities that really do shift the way you see the world.

Jane, one of my practice members amazed me with her level of gratitude and its healing power a while ago. While we were having a conversation about gratitude during her adjustment, she shared something profound with me. Jane's husband had passed away many years ago when their daughter was very young. As a widower and a single parent, Jane told me that she was actually grateful for that massive challenge. She had reached a point of gratitude for the death of her partner: she could now actually say thank you to her deceased husband for giving her the gift of being a single mother and experiencing being a parent from all aspects. That's how powerful gratitude can be.

Without gratitude we see life in an unbalanced way where the world is against you and you're the victim of the tides and the currents of the world, stumbling from one crisis to another. You'll have mood swings, you'll have a short temper, you'll have more low moods than not and you'll have a gloomy picture of your life ahead of you. You might feel stuck or blocked or frustrated and that there's no way forward for you. Such frustration can build up into anger and disappointment with your current situation. You feel no real drive or motivation to make the changes necessary or if you do, you simply don't have the energy, the ability or the willpower to maintain these changes. Your body is in defence physiology and that may lead your body to hold onto fat, especially around your belly, and could stop you from gaining lean muscle mass. It will prime you for injury and pain, lock up your movement and give you low energy and drive. It will rob you of your natural radiance and even create hormone imbalances in your body.

When you cultivate a state of gratitude you achieve a state of mental and physical balance – homeostasis – within your body. Your immune system is stronger, you'll have an improved hormonal balance. You'll increase those hormones associated with slowing the ageing process. You'll have faster recovery. You'll have an upwelling of positive emotions and you'll be more balanced in this mental state with a brighter outlook on life. You'll be more adaptable to change around you. You'll be able to better respond to challenges. You'll have a greater feeling of connection. You'll have improved levels of well-being. You'll feel greater satisfaction in your life. Frustration, anger and disappointment will dissolve as you rise above them and find new resources and new answers to more important questions.

In my experience gratitude has been a key factor in people's physical results too. Once they accept who they are and what they look like they begin to feel better about themselves. They immediately start acting in new ways and seeing new possibilities. With a sense of gratitude for who you are you can take actions steps you never thought possible. The key to this process is to practise this habit every day in a quiet setting. Just five minutes a day is all it will take to get started.

Learn from the pro's
What many people try to do is to think positively during a period of high emotional stress during the day. That's almost impossible unless you've practised it, because your brain isn't in a state to accept that information when it's in defence. It's like a tennis player practising a new serving technique during the finals of Wimbledon. It just doesn't happen. They would have to do that off court for hours on end to be able to put it into practise during the heat of the match. We need practise so we can grow new connections for gratitude in our brain every day in order to have the tools to adapt during the times of stress.

The hardest part of this daily exercise is simply waking up five minutes earlier! I recommend you do this in the morning five minutes before everybody else wakes up because that's when you're guaranteed to get some quiet time. In my experience, people who try and do it during the day often find it tough because of distractions and might not practise as consistently as they want. Because other things get in the way as other people's priorities might influence your day, waking up five minutes earlier creates your own priority time and you're guaranteed to get some quiet time to do this exercise.

Since our brains are powerful at doing pattern-recognition, once we prime them to find these patterns of gratitude we'll begin to see opportunities and solutions emerge around us. When this happens you begin to transcend those old beliefs so that you can develop new ones.

Creating a gratitude journal of all the things you're grateful for is a great way to begin this shift. It'll also serve as a reminder of how extraordinary your life really is, even when you're feeling uninspired. Practising in the morning, you'll be programming your mind to look for things to be grateful for. You'll begin to see new perspectives on challenges and opportunities that come your way with a different frame of mind and you'll be more productive. You'll feel more connected to the people around you.

Play

Play is the highest form of research.
ALBERT EINSTEIN

In *The Primal Connection*, Mark Sisson states, "Play nurtures our creative energies and strengthens our problem solving skills. For tens of thousands of years, it was a vital component of communal living and social cohesion among our hunter-gatherer ancestors."

Play is a luxury for children in our human zoo; it's something we afford children and frown on for adults. When children have no time in their busy schedules for free, unstructured, leisurely play we know we have a problem.

Playfulness is a gift that is innate to each of us from birth. We use play to learn how to navigate the world of social interaction. We use it to learn new things about the physical world around us and we use it to learn new things, like languages.

As a baby you would never have been able to progress from lying down to rolling over, to sitting up, to crawling, to walking and on to running without having a sense of play about it. Somewhere along the line we forgot how to play, or play was programmed out of us as we grew up. Through school or university and definitely through work we get told that play is unimportant. Play, however, is something we're genetically programmed to do and without it we're not going to grow and repair anymore; we're going to defend and decay.

Play is how we most effectively learn. When we are working on those things that are of highest value to ourselves it doesn't feel like work, it feels like we're playing, like we're doing something enjoyable, and we can reach amazing heights. This is how people win Nobel Prizes! They do something they enjoy and it takes them onto newer and higher levels with newer innovations, insights and meanings. The same skill of play that takes a child from crying to babbling to talking is the same process that takes us to human ingenuity and genius.

Looking at our lifestyle right now, though, we have a distinct play deficit. Children growing up now have so much of their time scheduled for specific extracurricular activities that there is simply no time or space in their schedule for unstructured play. Even the sports field where play could flourish is often taken so seriously that there is very little sense of fun in it anymore. We could be playing a sport for enjoyment and instead it has become a must-win task.

Through active learning you keep your brain young, you keep it growing and repairing. By learning you're stimulating new parts of the brain to grow, remould and redevelop. You keep your brain young and you stave off any mental decline that is common in old age. This decline is absolutely not your genetic destiny. Play is a critical key to your learning. How about being more connected with the people around you and being able to navigate social situations with ease and grace and lightness? This all comes down to a sense of play.

We might watch a two year old take a toy away from another child and see them crying. What invariably happens is that parents intervene and say, "No, that's bad." We could be leaving them to sort it out themselves through play. If we let them figure it out they might learn that if we take a toy away from another kid it's going to make them unhappy and they're not going to want to play with us. This is how we learn to share. By making mistakes we learn and play in a safe environment.

We learn the rules of social situations as children through play. When parents hover over our children they're programming play out of them. The children are losing that connection, that natural ability to grow and learn and develop and integrate insights and meanings from many different situations through play. The best way to learn is through play.

How about bonding with the people closest to you? The people that you tend to have the most fun with are the people that you feel closest to. In an age where we're becoming increasingly isolated from people and we're getting more and more artificial interactions instead of real authentic human interaction, being playful is probably one of the most powerful things we can do to reconnect and to integrate with our own social circle and in society as a whole.

From my experience I've noticed that those people who age better biologically, mentally and emotionally tend to be the most playful, the most curious, the most fun loving, the most mischievous. There's something about a state of curiosity that changes our biological ageing process and helps us to grow and repair for longer and so helps us to enjoy life longer. To activate growth and repair, to live a life of vitality it's important that we foster that sense of curiosity in life, that sense of play, that sense of fun.

So what is play, exactly? Stuart Brown, author of *Play: How it Shapes the Brain, Opens the Imagination and Invigorates the Soul* says play will be many different things to different people. To some play might be gardening, while to others it might be playing sports. *What* it is isn't as important as *how* we do it. He lists the following properties of play and they are elements that you can incorporate into your life and your transformation:

- **PURPOSELESS** – there is no real aim or goal in sight. This is why you tend to believe that play is a waste of time but it's also exactly why you need it. When you release the outcome you open yourself to opportunity.
- **VOLUNTARY** – play is fun and that makes it attractive. When you really let your hair down, everyone wants to play and you can't be bored when you play.
- **FREEDOM FROM TIME** – when you are fully engaged in play you lose your sense of passage of time and your consciousness of self diminishes. You let go and aren't afraid to look silly. This is similar to being in 'the zone' or what Mihaly Csikszentmihalyi calls 'flow'.
- **IMPROVISATIONAL POTENTIAL** – in play you are open to serendipity and chance. You let go of rules and restrictions and have the chance to see things from new angles and discover new ways of being.
- **CONTINUATION DESIRE** – the pleasure of the experience of play drives your desire to continue playing.

When I first read this list I thought that it was nice but was reserved for children or 'non-productive' members of society. But as I observe the world around me I often found that people who were happy and successful seemed to be playing all the time. They seemed fearless at work and not afraid to make mistakes, learn from them and move on; they seemed to have boundless energy and enthusiasm to keep going. Many of them didn't seem self-conscious at all. They would put themselves out there and do silly things but people wouldn't laugh at them because they were laughing with them.

A lack of play is a deficiency of the signals our genes expect. Any deficiency to our genetic expectation is a stressor and stressors unbalance our mind-body and lead us to defence and decay.

Since that realisation I have been conscious of frequently bringing play into my life. In the office we even have a policy that states that we don't work, we 'play with purpose'. ●

> *The why is the shining, golden thread that guides is,*
> *compels us and inspires us to take the next step*
> *and the one after that and the one after that.*
> *One step, one choice at a time we transform,*
> *we become and we manifest our future selves.*
> DAN MILLERMAN

11

Eat real food

Rule 1.
Rule 2.
That is all.

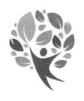

A philosophy of food

Diets do not work but a change in diet is definitely a requirement for a healthy lifestyle. This is one of the biggest conundrums facing people who are looking to improve their health. The cause of the problem is not poor eating, that's just a symptom. The cause of the problem is a poor relationship with food. To improve our nutrition and our health we must heal our relationship with food.

Healing your relationship with food means having some awareness of what real food is and what it isn't. Where real food comes from and how best to prepare and eat real food. You don't have to become a farmer, a chef or a nutritionist, but you do have to become aware.

What is food to you? Is it simply fuel or is it a source of comfort too? Do you use food to celebrate or to connect with people? Do you show your love by feeding people? It pays to become aware of your own beliefs around nutrition by being mindful of your relationship with food.

How did wild free humans eat?

Now we come to nutrition, that most emotive of topics that everyone has an opinion on. Before going ahead here recall the story of the blind men with the elephant. Each of them had a piece of the truth but none had a full idea of the elephant. The many factions of the nutritional world, from vegans to low-carb-high-fat adherents, have some justification of their views based on their experience and their view of science. We're not claiming to have *the answer*; this is not the end of the debate but we do believe that we have a much bigger view and a very useful starting point.

We are aiming for a vitalisitc lifestyle that helps you live a bigger life. We're not aiming to find a diet that gets you the fastest weight loss. We're looking for the way of eating that provides full and sufficient nutrients to your mind-body, one that eliminates toxicities and deficiencies. We're looking for the way of life that stimulates growth and repair on a cellular level, allowing your mind-body to shed excess fat, improve moods and energy, boost focus, improve strength, balance hormones, improve immune function and help us to fulfil your human potential.

Diet is a topic that can and does consume whole books and since this is not another diet book I'm not going to delve into the fine detail very deeply, and that's a good thing. It's a good thing because it's useful to give you perspective – an overview of the template so you can learn some of the principles from an aerial view and not get confused by different people's interpretation of what happens on the ground. You can use the tools we give you for yourself and then decide if you think it does what we say it does. Remember, we're looking for useful heuristics.

Wild free humans ate a very broad range of food that was available to them and different groups had access to different foods. In the search for common patterns though there are consistent similarities.

Many of the foods that they ate are no longer available to us. Like Mokolo's zoo keepers who couldn't get the exact same plants as his wild cousins in Rwanda, we're going to approximate and use what we do have. We aren't looking to recreate history here; we're using it as a template.

So, what was on the menu? Well, our wild free humans were definitely omnivores, that much is certain, so meat, fish, foul, eggs, plants in the form of fruit, vegetables, honey and some nuts and seeds are all on the menu. They ate what was seasonally available and everything was definitely locally sourced and organic.

Contrast that with the average westerner's diet and there is a stark difference. As hunter-gatherers, there was obviously nothing pre-packaged or processed with additives and preservatives.

Grains and legumes were rarely eaten, if at all, because there were no ways to cultivate or process them. Dairy was not on the menu as cows or goats hadn't been domesticated yet and trying to milk a wild beast is not a good idea if you value your life. Vegetable oils were non-existent neither was anything with processed sugar or preservatives and alcohol wasn't around yet.

I said that we don't want to recreate history by eating *exactly* what they used to eat; we couldn't if we tried. Many plants that were around then are no longer here and many of our staple foods, like broccoli, are more recent farming inventions so that's not the point.

Instead of plodding down the aisles in a supermarket filling our trolley with food-like substances, what we can do is take what we know about what wild free humans ate and determine guidelines that will help us navigate our Neolithic supermarkets and farmers markets more gracefully. When we do this we come up with two rules.

RULE 1: Food quality

Eat real, biologically appropriate food that was recently living
A lion doesn't eat what a giraffe does, nor does a gorilla eat what a tiger does. When given the choice, each animal will stick to their biologically appropriate foods and these foods will not only sustain them but allow them to thrive. This simple principle tells us that the nutrition of each species is specific to each species.

A lion in South Africa will eat the same type of food as a lion in Kenya and the same is true for giraffes in those different locations. Though the exact foods may differ the type will be the same. For example the giraffes of Kenya may have access to and eat the leaves of a slightly different tree than in South Africa, but they won't be eating leaves in one place and the monkeys in the trees in the other.

Just like Mokolo the gorilla got sick when he ate foods that were not biologically appropriate and started to get better once he was moved to food more appropriate for his physiology, so too do humans have the same reaction.

Foods exist on a spectrum from high to low quality. The quality is judged by how biologically appropriate the food is and whether the animal can get the nutrients from this food and not be harmed by the toxins. Artificially formulated gorilla biscuits are low quality for gorillas while fresh produce is higher quality.

Low quality foods might be able to keep you alive but not without paying a price. Low quality foods come with low grade toxins that your physiology can't deal with. These foods damage you, sometimes very slowly, and cause our bodies to go into survival mode and create defence physiology. Over time defence becomes decay with chronic inflammation and that leads to disease.

Obesity, diabetes, heart disease, cancer, depression, chronic fatigue, chronic pain, IBS, ADHD, acne and osteoporosis are just some examples of the conditions that low quality food can contribute to. By the time you realise you are in the disease phase, there is already a significant amount of damage done and it will take time to heal properly if you don't already have some degree of permanent damage.

High quality food nourishes and protects your mind and body. High quality food deflames your ecosystem sends the cells of your body into thrive mode. From your liver to your brain, your heart to your lungs and everything besides, they begin with growth and repair. Over time growth and repair can regenerate your body and lead you to experience vitality.

There are many remarkable stories and some compelling scientific studies detailing how moving to more natural and ancestral patterns of eating can and does transform lives and help many health issues. I've witnessed many first hand. It's important to stress here that this way of eating is *not* a treatment for any condition or disease but a way of helping your mind-body most effectively activate growth and repair.

Those same issues that poor nutrition can play a part in creating, a vitalistic lifestyle can play a part in healing.

Food Tests: (adapted from *It Starts with Food* by Dallas and Melissa Hart)
We can test foods on four standards of how they affect our physiology. High quality foods will pass four of these tests, while low quality foods will fail one or more.

1. **Mental test**
   We've evolved over millions of years to be drawn to certain tastes because they were associated with highly nutritious foods. In nature, the pleasure we would have derived from consuming these foods would have been followed by the vital nutrition they packed, so we're wired to be drawn to these foods.

   Because you have a natural attraction to these tastes, you are also vulnerable to letting your senses be hijacked by excessive amounts, or artificial sources, of these foods, which causes us to over consume them. Foods failing this test fit in to the category of superstimulus or food porn.

   The theory of hyperpalatability has good research behind it and says that one of the main causes of obesity and it's related health issues is our weakness to superstimulating foods.

   Some foods can cause problems in your appetite control centres of the brain called your appestat by causing hormone imbalances and affecting your reward pathways deep in your brain. When this happens you might feel hungry all the time and you will crave certain tastes.

2. Hormonal test

Food is meant to help you to get to and stay in growth and repair mode. That means it will create a balanced metabolism leading to a balanced mind-body. Foods that disrupt that balance and cause hormone imbalance, resistance or over-sensitivity will move you from growth and repair to defence and decay.

Certain hormones play key roles in influencing your appestat and if the foods and drinks we take in cause derangement to the balance of those hormones our appetite and cravings will get the best of us. Leptin, ghrelin and neuropeptide Y are examples of these hormones.

3. Gut test

Not only does it digest and absorb our food but about 80% of your immune system calls the gut home, so you really want to keep it happy. Your gut is the thing that stands in the way of getting waste (poo) into your bloodstream. You want to maintain the integrity of our gut.

The happiness of your gut is intimately connected with your gut microbiome made up of all the bacteria, viruses and parasites that dwell within us. These organisms have likely shaped much of our evolution. Our understanding of the microbiome is very limited right now and we do know that the foods we eat heavily influence which type of microscopic life-form is calling us home.

Damage to the gut has been linked to brain degeneration, mood and behavioural issues, arthritis, chronic pain, obesity, cancers, every type of autoimmune condition, heart disease and even diabetes (type 1 and 2).

4. Immune system and inflammatory test

Real foods will strengthen and sustain your immune system. They'll allow it to be prepared and effective when needed but keep it in the background when it's not needed, like your personal attack dog.

Letting the dog off the leash and allowing it to attack everything including ourselves is not a good idea and can result in chronic inflammation that can ravage us from the inside, playing a causal role in cancers, heart disease, depression, obesity and all autoimmune conditions.

RULE 2: Nutrient density

Nourish your mind-body with every mouthful.
When we're living lives that are more stressful than ever, why would we not want to maximise our nutrition?

Why would we not want the most bang for our buck with every mouthful of food and with every cent we spend on that food?

We live in times where we put incredible strain on our mind-body and yet our food is very nutrient poor. Conventional farming practices deplete our soil of nutrients which are then further spoiled by refining and processing.

Many of the very common conditions that seem to afflict us are actually problems of malnutrition. In order to nourish our mind-body we need to be consuming foods that have the maximum amount of nutrients in them.

There is no time to waste on foods that are poor in nutrients; that's like filling up your car with a filler instead of petrol. You're spending time and money filling up your tank, so maximise your investment with quality fuel.

Foods put to the test

Junk fodder
Crisps, sweets, snacks, fizzy drinks, ready meals, take-aways... we're not even going to call this stuff food. If you're following these principles it's clear that it's best to eliminate all junk. This highly processed, low quality, low nutrient density fodder acts like drugs to make you crave them and they damage your body. These 'Franken-foods' come in packaging and range from pre-prepared microwave meals to snacks and sweets.

They fail all four food standards. They can punch holes in your gut, inflame your system, create hormonal imbalances, distort sugar balances, shrink your brain and shred your arteries and much, much more.

With all this damage happening, your body has to do defence and decay. Remember defence and decay means you can't do growth and repair. No growth and repair means your personal performance is dampened, energy is lower, focus is fuzzier, weight-loss impaired, immune system is impeded and you're more susceptible to disease.

FOOD STANDARDS FAILED
1   2   3   4

Grains – poverty food:

Grains are such a cheap commodity, produced in such vast quantities that they can be called the darling of the food industry. For very little cost they can be used in many products and give a good profit margin. Unfortunately, foods based on them are usually of a very low quality food with many ill-effects. Wheat is the most common grain and probably the worst – maize, millet, barley, spelt, rye, oats and rice are others.

Refined or unrefined, some grains have more problems than others. Many grains, wheat chief among them, can hijack your reward pathways and cause you to over consumer them. Anyone who has had the jitters at the thought of giving up bread will know what I mean.

When it comes to bread and pasta I've found many people I work with have trouble letting them go. If this is you, here is a good way to think of it. When you're eating a sandwich or some pasta – it's the filling of the sauce that you're after. Ditch the starchy glue and just have more of the filling!

Through their antinutrients, enzyme inhibitors and low-grade toxins like gluten they contribute to a host of issues that don't just affect your gut: from bloating, constipation and diarrhoea to skin problems to chronic pain to brain, nerve and mood issues, grains are likely suspects. They have been strongly linked to autoimmune diseases (like multiple sclerosis, rheumatoid arthritis, thyroid deficiency, colitis) and affects all organs including the gut, the brain, the liver and the thyroid.

This means that even though things like oats are technically gluten free, they might still be irritants and can also be excluded by cutting out grains completely. Even small doses of grains can cause damage that can last weeks to months. See the list *Grains in Disguise* to find out where grains and grain products have been hidden in your foods.

Grains also fail the hormone standard, mainly because they cause a release of blood sugar very quickly, some faster than table sugar itself. After repeated bouts of this sugar onslaught your body no longer responds to hormones like insulin and leptin the way it should and hormone resistance ensues. Now we have discord in our hormonal symphony and everything from brain to reproductive function is compromised. While rice may not be a strong gut irritant it does deliver a big load of starch that is rapidly converted into sugar.

Grains promote chronic inflammation in the body through their effect on the immune system, gut and hormones.

Grains are also very low in nutrient density (yes, even whole grains) when compared to biologically appropriate foods like meat, fish, foul, eggs and vegetables. They are generally not worthy of inclusion in our lifestyle.

FOOD STANDARDS FAILED
1   2   3   4

Pseudo-grains and sprouted grains:
Buckwheat, chia, quinoa, coxcomb, goosefoot, wattleseed and amaranth are not quite the same as grains and are called pseudo-grains. They represent a better choice than grains like wheat and maize but they may not be innocent foods.

Grains and pseudo-grains that are soaked and allowed to sprout are also potentially better choices. This is a time consuming process though and it's not certain whether soaking, sprouting or even fermenting them really tames all of their harmful nature.

While the scientific jury is out on exactly how these affect us, those of us who are battling conditions and food sensitivities would do well to avoid them.

Sugars – food heroin:
Cheap and nasty, that's the best way to describe sugar. It comes in a few forms and all of them are worth eliminating from your life. Added sugars are highly processed products, often tainted with chemicals from their creation process.

These sugars affect your mind-body in a myriad of ways from setting off chronic stress responses and creating chronic inflammation, to disabling your immune system to fuelling cancer cells. Add into the mix their addictive nature and you can realise their potential to wreak havoc with your health.

If that wasn't enough, sugar also causes hormone imbalances and resistance, promotes fat storage and affects muscle building. Sugars play havoc with your concentration, memory and moods too.

What about sugar free sweeteners like aspartame, saccharin, sucralose, stevia and xylitol? These are chemicals that have a sweet taste and are best avoided. What most people aren't aware of is that the sweet taste these chemicals produce can create the same physiological cascade in your body and set off the same harmful effects to your mind-body that sugar does. Sweeteners also damage your gut because they are linked to imbalanced gut bacteria and keep your palate used to the supernormal stimulus of sweetened foods.

Natural fruit sugar (fructose) is acceptable if it comes with the whole fruit. Juicing does not count unless you do it at home and include all of the pulp, too. Without all the pulp fruit juice is a concentrated fructose hit that is closer to refined sugar than a nutrient.

Some sugars are strongly linked with cancer and other diseases and are marketed as 'natural sugar replacements.' They are all heavily processed and it's a good idea to avoid all of them.

FOOD STANDARDS FAILED
1   2   3   4

Seed oils – bad fats:
From canola oil to corn oil, peanut oil to sunflower oil, these chemicals are definitely worth eliminating from your life. We're not even classing these as foods; they are industrial chemicals badly disguised as food. Margarine is a clear culprit here too that is best excluded.

Seed oils are processed at high temperatures and created with toxic chemicals like petrochemicals, bleaches, acids and deodorisers, many of which can't be fully removed from the final product. They are laced with damaging trans-fats and are important to remove from your diet.

These oils cause chronic inflammation, affect your immune system, disrupt normal cell function, scupper weight loss and can affect your brain too. Do you really want to be eating these chemicals?

FOOD STANDARDS FAILED
2   4

Dairy – cow's breast milk:
Can you think of an animal that breastfeeds off another animal into adulthood? I've asked this question to many biologists and none have been able to give me an answer other than humans. Cow's milk is good for calves, it is biologically appropriate for them just as human milk is biologically appropriate for human babies. It contains all the hormones, enzymes, sugars, fats, immune complexes and proteins that the calf needs to double its weigh in about 49 days. That's what cow's milk is for. Would you feed human breast milk to a calf?

Dairy is in essence a growth promoter for baby cows. It triggers hormonal cascades that have far reaching consequences. The proteins in dairy (whey and casein) seem to have the strongest effect here. They have the potential to get through the gut and trigger hormonal responses that compromise our own hormonal symphony. The sugar in dairy (lactose) can also disturb our hormones.

Dairy is not biologically appropriate for humans, especially when you consider that, under conventional farming practices, hormones and antibiotics are added, good fats are removed during homogenisation and pasteurisation destroys many nutrients that might have been in the milk initially. Low fat and skim dairy products are particularly low quality foods.

Pasture raised cattle allowed to feed on grass that are free from hormones and antibiotics may produce milk of a higher quality. If this is consumed raw and unprocessed then there may be some nutrient value that could be useful and so this is a very grey area. Questions of food safety and hygiene exist so it's best to avoid dairy if you can't be sure of where it's come from.

FOOD STANDARDS FAILED
2

A note on meat

Meat is an essential source of nutrition that our mind-body expects. So while eating meat from fish, game, poultry, cows, pigs and many other animals is biologically appropriate, animal cruelty in the form of mass production of flesh of all kinds is detrimental to your health and that of our greater ecosystem. Are the animals that you eat pasture-reared or free range and allowed to eat their natural diet? Or are they confined to pens in which they can't move and forced to consume feed to bulk them up while being injected with all manner of hormones and antibiotics? Were they treated well and slaughtered in a humane way? Just remember you are what you eat. You are also what you eat has eaten, and you are how it was treated.

Be a label expert

All your good intentions may come undone if you don't arm yourself with some tools to combat the sneaky practices of many food manufacturers. Learn their tricks.

Grains in disguise:

Wheat, wheat flour, bran flour, germ, wheat germ, whole wheat flour, enriched flour, hydrolysed wheat/plant/plant protein, texturised vegetable protein, hydrogenated vegetable protein, MSG, maltodextrin, dextrin, edible starch, binders, stabilisers, natural flavours, barley, rye, spelt.

Pay special attention to sauces (including soy sauce) and beers.

Sugar in disguise:

Sugar, cane/rice/palm/corn sugar, high fructose corn syrup (HFCS), maize syrup, dextrose, fructose, glucose, lactose, hydrogenated starch, modified starch, malt, malted barley/maize, maltodextrin, mannitol, agave, ethyl maltol, sorbitol, caramel.

Remember to look out for sweeteners like aspartame, saccharin, sucralose, stevia and xylitol!

BOTTOM LINE:
Nutrients – high quality foods:

Meat, fish, fowl, eggs, vegetables, fruit, some nuts and seeds and herbs and spices: these foods are in their whole food state (like they've just come off the farm) and are eaten as fresh as possible.

Toxins – low quality foods:

Grains (wheat, maize, rye, barley, spelt, oats, millet, rice), legumes (beans, peanuts, chickpeas, cashews), dairy, vegetable oils and sugars (including alcohol).

RULE OF THUMB:
Anything in a packet with more than three ingredients
is assumed to be process or refined.

ELIMINATING TOXINS

Supernormal stimulus: human kryptonite

Franken-foods like sweeteners, colorants, flavourings, MSG, corn syrup and seed oils are the main culprits here; they fail the mental food standard. They are cheap to produce and overwhelm your rational willpower by hijacking the hardwired reward pathways in your brain. They can create dependency similar to that of cocaine or heroine.

Luckily, they are easy to avoid. Most packaged foods that have names that sound more like chemicals than food are likely to be human kryptonite. Simply steer clear of food in a package that has three or more ingredients in it.

Now that food scientists have figured out our evolutionary Achilles heel, they have been able to manipulate the tastes of processed foods to play on our weakness. Every processed food will use a combination of sweet, salty, fatty and umami tastes to hook you while providing plenty of toxins and little if any of the nutritional value your body expects.

These chemicals are also suspected of being involved in gut damage, cancers, heart disease and obesity. They can affect brain function and disrupt your hormonal balance. Steer clear of all of them.

Biologically appropriate nutrition

High quality, nutrient dense foods:

Source organic and pasture raised foods where possible.

Quality ⟶

Nutrients

MODERATION CHOICES:
Eat and drink in moderation

**Fruit, nuts and seeds,
starchy vegetables ...**

WISE CHOICES:
Eat and drink to satiety
'Smart, slim and youthful'

**Meat, fish, fowl, eggs,
non-starchy vegetables,
herbs and spices**

Toxins

ILL-ADVISED CHOICES:
Shun these foods and drinks
'Stupid, fat and decrepit'

**Grains, sugars, seed oils,
legumes, conventional dairy,
alcohol ...**

QUESTIONABLE CHOICES:
Avoid these second rate foods

**Raw dairy, pseudo-grains and
some beans and legumes ...**

Nutrient Density ⟶ *Source fresh produce as much as possible.*

Foods exist on a spectrum from high to low quality and from high to low nutrient density. If we plot different types of foods into their categories then we come up with a Food Matrix.

Food table

Protein	Vegetables Non	Fats		Herbs and Spices	
Chicken	Cabbage	Coconut Oil	HIgh heat cooking and frying	Mint	Salt
Beef	Broccoli	Lard		Coriander	Tarragon
Pork	Cauliflower	Ghee		Dill	Basil
Lamb	Peppers (red, green and yellow)	Palm Oil		Oregano	Chives
Fish	Asparagus	Clarified Butter		Parsley	Clove
Shell fish	Leafy greens	Butter	Browning and sautéing at lower temps	Garlic	Fennel
Eggs	Carrots	Normal Olive Oil		Ginger	Horseradish
Game (kudu, ostrich, springbok, etc.)	Parsnip	Nut Oils	Flavour food after cooking	Lemon Grass	Bay Leaf
Liver, sweetbread, kidney, etc.	Onion	Avocado Oil		Allspice	Lemon/Lime
	Acocado	High quality extra virgin olive oil		Chilli	Saffron
	Kale			Tumeric	Vanilla
	Pumpkin			Cinnamon	Watercress
	Swuash			Paprika	Lavender
	Sweet Potato			Cumin	
	Yam			Pepper	
	Celery			Rosemary	
	Cucumber			Curry	
	Brussel sprout			Cardamon	
	Pak Choy			Mustard	
	Raddish				
	Artichoke				
	Tomato				

Eliminating toxins

Your life without sugar, grains, legumes, dairy and vegetable oils.
Since the toxins we've listed are ubiquitous in modern diets, some people feel at a complete loss when they try to remove them. Others claim that they get bored if they just stick to the list of nutrients.

To help with mental block we've created a Food Table that you can use to create around 61000 meals! The table is a good starting place. It is not a complete and definitive list of all that is and all that is not biologically appropriate.

> To get a downloadable copy of the Food Table to print out and put on your fridge, go to http://THRIVElifestyle.solutions/food-table

How much do I eat?
If you stick to the nutrients we listed and eliminate the toxins you should be able to eat until you are full at every meal, provided you eat in 'High Definition' as described in the Action Steps section.

If you find you are hungry and need to snack between meals you may be eating too little food or may be taking in low quality or nutrient sparse foods that are affecting your appestat.

What about calories?
The truth is that we are very bad at calculating the calories in foods and the way your body is going to use those calories is very different from the way mine will. Food labelling for calories is all based on 19th century laboratory experiments that have been called into question.

Start with the food itself. Not all apples will have the same amount of calories and even two of the same type grown in different places will differ.

Next we need to look at how the processing of the food, whether it is cooking, soaking, sprouting or fermenting in your own home or industrially refining, enhancing, preserving or otherwise altering your food it changes how many calories you can extract.

Digestion is the next step and this is a very complex, not to mention messy process. How your gut works on foods and how mine does can be very different and your food labels don't take any of that into account.

The composition of your gut microbiome is another dizzyingly complex confounding factor. Which bacteria are present and active will make a significant difference to how you digest you food. This bacterial balance will also change in response to the food you eat so your digestion might be different on different days.

Once you've digested your food, how you use it will differ too. While fats carry more calories than carbohydrates and proteins, they are all used for far more than just energy. Fats make up your cell walls while proteins are the building blocks of muscles. A type of carbohydrate called fibre is not digested well but can be used to feed your gut bacteria. You have no idea how your body is going to use the calories you consume. Eat real food and get on with living your life.

Are carbs bad?
Remember Rule 1? Fresh vegetables and fruits are high quality foods that contain carbohydrate and we want to include them in our diet. Rule 2 says that we want to have nutrient dense foods and vegetables have a good nutrient density while fruits are generally average.

Some hunter-gatherers ate up to 60% of their calories as carbs on a seasonal basis and had no obesity while some had much less. Interestingly none of them were zero carb if they could help it.

Technically speaking what we're avoiding are called *acellular* carbohydrates. These are carbs that have had their starch freed from its cellular cage. This makes them volatile in our body. Think refined flours, fruit juices and pulverised dried fruit bars.

Our approach will be lower in carbs than the average western diet because we are excluding grains, most starchy carbs and processed foods, but it's not necessarily a 'very low carb' diet (aka Banting, Atkins or LCHF).

Low-carb-high-fat (LCHF) approaches can be very useful, often result in dramatic weight loss and improvement of health and are used as treatments for specific conditions. I've used them myself with great success.

What's not clear though is whether they get to the cause of the problem, which is damaged glucose metabolism and is strongly linked to chronic inflammation.

Promising lines of research to address the issue of glucose metablism include managing your alloststic load, improving your physical strength and conditioning, learning to balance mental and emotional stress, improving sleep and recovery and addressing your gut microbiome.

If you would like to be low carb while living a vitalistic lifestyle them simply avoid fruits and include in non-starchy vegetables.

What about carbs for energy?

What most people don't realise is that your body can run on carbs or fat as a fuel source. The difference is that we burn fats cleaner than we burn carbs and it is possible to become 'fat adapted' so that your body preferentially burns fat as a energy source.

What about fats, cholesterol and heart disease?

It's been repeated so many times over the years that eating saturated fat causes heart disease because of its effect on cholesterol. While we've been living in a world where conventional wisdom has accepted 'low-fat' as healthy, it might surprise you to learn however, after many years of research, we've learned that saturated fat has less of an effect on heart health than you think and that cholesterol is a vital nutrient in your body.

Cholesterol is a very important chemical in our bodies; every cell in your body needs it to stay alive, it forms the basis of hormones, vitamins, it works in repair of cells, it is a major constituent of your brain, it helps you fight infection and much, much more.

Where there is some link between cholesterol and heart disease revolves around chronic inflammation. So it's not the cholesterol that's the issue it's the damage inflammation does to it that could be problematic.

Good fats *vs* bad fats?

Good fats are listed in the Food Table and also include those from animal sources when the animals have been allowed to eat their natural food and have been raised in good conditions.

A good example is the fat in fresh, wild caught fish. It is very healthful and loaded with omega 3! A piece of sirloin with the fat on from a grass-fed cow is also high in omega 3.

If we feed cows on grains (like maize or oats), which are not biologically appropriate for them, then we start running into trouble, so leaner cuts of these lower quality meats are advised.

Fats in the form of oils from nuts can be useful, as long as the oil can be extracted without extensive processing, which would break Rule 1. Look for cold pressed or 'virgin' oils.

It's useful here to look at the label once again. Make sure the oil hasn't been processed, deodorised or chemically altered.

What about supplements?
Think of supplements like decorations in a house. They may help to make the place feel better for you but without a strong foundation and walls, they are next to useless. It's far more useful to ensure your foundation is sound before you decorate your walls. The foundation here is your lifestyle and you can't out supplement a poor lifestyle.

Many people become sidetracked by supplements and miss out on some of the nutritional fundamentals that are far more helpful. They spend lots of money on the next new 'superfood' and never get the basics sorted out. While their pocket is lightened their health and human potential suffers.

Most supplements are expensive urine makers at best and potentially dangerous at worst. Only supplement with nutrients that are biologically appropriate and that your whole food diet is deficient in.

Meal replacement shakes and formulas are not real food and do not address the real problem, which is your relationship with food. These products are highly refined and are no match for eating real food that was recently living.

Biologically appropriate supplementation:
Supplement with nutrients you require for health and that you cannot get from whole food sources.

THE BIG THREE INCLUDE:

- **Omega 3 fish oils** – our balance of omega fatty acids in our body is dangerously imbalanced in most industrialised societies. We tend to have too much Omega 6 and too little Omega 3. You can get this from food sources like fresh cold-water fish and grass fed meat though they usually carry a higher price tag. Vegetarian sources of Omega 3 are not used well in our bodies.
- **Probiotics** – we are exposed to a vastly reduced load of microorganisms now than at any other point in our evolution. While that has been useful in some aspects we may have gone too far. By over sterilising our environment we have become deficient and imbalanced in our exposure to bacteria, viruses, fungi and parasites. As much as we're taught to fear these guys (and sometimes for good reason) the truth seems to be that we are evolved to live with them and that they are part of a vitalistic lifestyle.
- **Vitamin D3** – our indoor lifestyle robs us exposure to the bright yellow star at the centre of our solar system. Rays from the sun are a nutrient that stimulates your mind-body to vitality, partly by helping us make our own Vitamin D. Sensible daily exposure to the sun without the use of sunscreens can help us make all the Vitamin D we need but since most of us don't get that, supplementation is necessary.

There may be other supplements that fit within our paradigm. I encourage you to search for whole food sources of things you may be deficient in before reaching for a supplement.

Without dairy, how do I get my calcium?

This is very common question and stems from the misinformation we've been fed for a long time. What we believe is that the strength of our teeth and bones is determined by how much calcium we eat. This has led to calcium supplements and medications being widely used with very limited effectiveness. These supplements have recently been linked with heart problems.

The truth is that there is much more that goes into making strong teeth and bones, like protein and Vitamin D. Calcium is important, but far more important than how much you eat is how much you can absorb and actually use.

On a biologically appropriate diet you will get a much better combination of the different elements, including calcium, to better nourish your body. Leafy greens, meats, seafood and bone broth are good sources of calcium that will give you enough to build and repair your teeth and bones.

If dairy is low quality, why is butter included?

Of the major issues dairy has, two stand out as particularly troublesome – milk sugar and milk protein. Heavy cream and butter are minimally processed and are virtually free of these troublesome compounds so they are useful in limited quantities.

Action steps

Shopping:
- Always shop on a full stomach.
- Find local farmers markets and buy local, seasonal food whenever possible.
- Only shop in the meat and fresh produce section and avoid the rest of the supermarket.
- Think of your trolley or basket as your body, anything you put in you'll most likely eat.
- Buy organic whenever possible. If cost is an issue then prioritise buying 'The Dirty Dozen' most pesticide laden foods as organic purchases.
- Anything in packaging with more than three ingredients is likely to be processed so put it down and move on.
- Be gluten free but don't buy 'gluten free'. Foods with these labels are going to be heavily refined and processed. Stick to real foods and ditch bread and pasta whatever their ingredients.

Preparing:
- Wash all fruits and vegetables thoroughly before cooking. A diluted apple cider vinegar solution is good for this.

Cooking:
- Use lower temperatures as much as possible and avoid burning foods.
- If frying or grilling at high temperatures, use the high heat oils on the food table.

Eating mindfully:
- **Start in a state of grace** – no matter your religious slant, take a moment to savour the sights and smells of your meal and be grateful for the nourishment it's about to provide you.

- **Eat in high definition** – Eat one mouthful at a time. Don't even prepare the next mouthful until you have finished the one you are on! This will help you to slow down, taste your food and get maximum pleasure from each mouthful.
- **Sit down to eat every meal,** no eating on the run, in your car or at your desk. ●

12

Move yourself

Why you love movement.
Stop exercising.
How a competent human moves.
Free your feet.
Play. Stop. Play.
Tribal wisdom.

Movement is a nutrient

Imagine we'd found a drug that could:

- Prevent up to 91% of cases of obesity and type 2 diabetes
- Prevent 50% of all cases of heart disease
- Reduce risk of stroke by 25-30%
- Prevent up to 50% of all stroke deaths
- Reduce congestive heart disease deaths by 63%
- Reduce hospital readmission for heart failure patients by 70%
- Normalise blood pressure and reduce risk of developing high blood pressure
- Restore or maintain heart and blood vessel health
- Restore and maintain normal cholesterol triglyceride levels
- Reduce risk of breast cancer by up to 60%
- Reduce pancreatic cancer in overweight people by 50%
- Reduce lung cancer, even in smokers, by 72%
- Reduce melanoma by over 72%
- Prevent up to 50% of colon cancer
- Reduce risk of developing and improve outcomes of rheumatoid arthritis and osteoarthritis
- Prevent osteoporosis and increase new bone formation
- Increase strength and balance
- Decrease gallbladder removal by 20% and decrease gallstones
- Improve digestion and decrease indigestion
- Improve bowel function and elimination
- Increase immune system function
- Increase anti-tumour activity and antioxidant levels
- Decrease all causes of mortality by 67% in the general population
- Decrease all causes of mortality by 50% in the 61-81 year olds
- Prevent up to 47% of cognitive impairment, prevent up to 63% of Alzheimer's and 52% of dementia
- Improve physical function in older adults
- Decrease chance of ever being in a nursing home
- Decrease rate of ageing
- Enhance learning by 12 times
- Increase dopamine and serotonin levels
- Decrease depression by 20%, including relapses
- Increase growth and healing hormones

- Decrease stress and body breakdown hormones
- Decrease body fat, obesity and weight gain

How much do you think that would be worth and how much do you think that would be marketed to you if we'd found a drug that could do all of these things? The amazing thing is these are the documented benefits of walking 30 minutes 3 times or more a week. This is incredibly important because it tells us, together with the epigenetics that we've looked at, that movement is not an optional thing in our life. Movement is a required nutrient for health. We know that movement alters 60% of your genes through epigenetics.

Walking for 30 minutes or more, 3 or more times a week is not a treatment for any of those conditions or diseases. It's not a treatment for cancer; it's not a treatment to make learning easier or better. Walking is a vital nutrient for expressing health and the absence of movement – the deficiency of movement – is what causes ill health conditions and diseases. Just as Vitamin C is a required nutrient for health, so is movement.

When you move you are sending signals to your mind-body that then changes the expression of up to 60% of your genes. That is massive, those genes then start all sorts of cellular functions that are associated with growth and repair and without them you are sending signals of defence and decay to your genes.

Movement is a fertiliser for our brain. If we don't move, we're robbing our brain of what it needs to be able to form new connections and keep growing and prevent it from ageing and decaying. Movement aids learning and balances minds. Many issues we see more and more commonly from ADHD to depression can have some deficiency of movement in their root cause.

We know movement helps to balance hormones. We know movement helps to move that delicate chemical dance in our body towards balance and growth, repair and vitality and we know that a lack of movement imbalances hormones.

We know movement helps us to have better bowel function and is incredibly important for gut health. Movement also improves your immune system, as well as preventing the chronic inflammation that shrinks your brain, shreds your arteries, cannibalises your muscles, leeches your bones and punches holes in your gut.

Movement affects your brain, your hormones and can affect your gut and your immune system, but all of those things also affect the structure of your body as well. What's important to realise is all of those systems affect each other as well. So this really is an ecosystem that we're dealing with and we know that the ecosystem is affected by how we eat and how we move, how we think and how subluxated we are and each of those things affects everything else.

Movement not exercise

The word exercise can have very negative connotations to many people. Maybe you were the fat kid in school; you were never good at sport, you didn't like the way you looked in your school physical education uniform or had a mean gym teacher. There could be any number of reasons you've decided you don't like exercise.

Exercise is 'weights and cardio'; it's a run, it's something contrived, forced, artificial and requires motivation from the outside-in. Exercise tends to be isolated, limited, repetitive, happens in a single plane, is mechanical, highly specialised and manufactured. You exercise to get a result like losing weight or getting strong. Think bicep curls, bench press, marathon running and cycling.

If exercising were the cure for our ills as it's touted to be then we would be a healthier species. Instead, the more exercise you do, the more unbalanced your mind-body becomes, the more defence and decay it does and the sicker you become.

What's more useful is to shift toward movement. Movement is innate to you, you were born to move. Movement is fun; movement happens spontaneously and can arrive anywhere. Movement uses many parts of the body through many dimensions, is functional, generalised, organic, creative and opportunistic. Movement happens because you love it. The side effect of movement is that it gives you results in body composition and strength, too.

Movement is biologically appropriate and encompasses what you might call exercise and includes what you do in your day-to-day life like climbing stairs, playing with your kids and carrying the shopping. It also includes having sex, tickle fights, dancing and playing with the dog. Movement is native to the outdoors whenever possible.

214

Movement is inspirational because there is a love for it inside each of us. Your mind-body delights in movement, your genes respond to it and your mind-body does growth, repair and balance within your life. When you focus on movement you make the world your playground and your field of mastery. You can move and play at the office just as much as you can in the gym. You can practise movement in the house and not only when on the road or on the field.

One of the biggest differences between exercise and movement is not in *what we do* but in *our intent*. Your intent is your why, your reason for doing something and your "Why" shapes your "How" and determines your "What". If you approach the gym as a playground to be discovered and explored, if you decide to be creative and express yourself physically in that space then it becomes movement to be practised and played, not exercise in the form of a workout.

Ditch the 'gym sessions' and 'workouts' and embrace play and practise. If you have a particular type of movement you enjoy, like running, lifting weights, yoga or CrossFit then I suggest you approach these as a form of play that you practise for mastery; become a student of your chosen movement.

Practise and play through movement is endlessly scalable. From the elderly to the ill and injured you can use the principles of movement to regain confidence and independence in your mind-body. From the young, to the enthusiasts to the hard-core amongst you, movement will boost your performance, broaden your base of physical competence and prevent injury.

This subtle but powerful shift in your perception of a physical activity can take it from something you do begrudgingly to something you do for joy. When we work on play and practise we open ourselves up to possibilities and pleasures. What new things can you discover when you play and what can you master as you practice?

Fit for life

Necessity meant that our wild, free humans were very active. They generally walked long distances each day, about 6 - 16km. Each day was different and there was variation in their movement. Some days were heavy lifting to build a shelter or carry a kill while others were a short walk for water or running in pursuit of a hunted animal. When they were active, they moved their bodies through many dimensions, across all ranges of motion, sometimes fast, sometimes slow, sometimes light and sometimes heavy. This variety led our ancestors to be generalists; they were all-round physically fit with competence in many areas of human movement.

Compare this with our days of sitting in offices interrupted with the occasional 'weights and cardio' approach to fitness. Firstly, we don't get nearly enough movement and, secondly, when we do move we don't get the variety or quality of movement our mind-body craves. This is a severe deficiency. If you wonder why your body is so tight, weak and easily injured then look no further.

The average fit person in industrialised society today is still an inferior physical specimen, lacking in strength, suffering stuck joints, poor cardiovascular fitness and prone to injury. The average wild, free human would give Olympic athletes a run for their money! Even hunter-gatherers in their 60's and 70's would have been physically active, productive members of society.

For an animal that is supposed to move every day, sitting for hours on end, year after year, atrophies your mind-body. We lose our freedom of movement, thought and expression. Creativity is dulled and we stew in a state of defence as we slowly decay while we live.

Wild, free humans had varied, full body, multidimensional movement, which gave them a good baseline of physical competence that not only enabled them to perform physically at high levels but also to avoid injuries.

By using movement you can once again reclaim the freedom in your mind-body that you've lost, and become fit for life. Being fit for life has a few meanings that are worth discussing here. The first is that you are fit for *life*; you aren't only fit when young and then let the excuse of old age rob you of freedom and confidence in your body. You have the capacity to be strong, fast, flexible and free well into your senior years.

Ray Clark felt like he was getting lazy at home after his wife of 67 years and his daughter passed away. So at the age of 98 he decided he would begin moving again. With the help of his 70 year old trainer he began to rediscover the joy of movement. At 102 years old Ray could row vigorously on a rowing machine and use kettle bells with the coordination of a much younger man.

Fit for life. That means we are able to physically navigate through life with grace. You can match the challenges that life throws at you by carrying heavy shopping bags, push starting a car, lifting and catching a heavy toddler and sprinting up the stairs all without straining yourself or risking injury well into your advanced years All of this is possible if we are clear and define fitness properly.

Broaden the base

Specialists are weak
Virtually all of the elite athletes I've had in my practices were very good at doing just one or two types of sports-specific activities. Like a formula 1 car performs well on a track but not off-road, these athletes can do amazing things in their discipline but their range of performance is very narrow. Put a triathlete on a touch rugby field and watch them get injured.

Endurance athletes, from elite to recreational, are especially prone to making this mistake. If running is a good thing to do then running more must be better, right? Well, it turns out that is wrong. 90% of people training for and running marathons get injured every year .

You are meant to be fit for life as a generalist first, with a broad base of physical competence, like a foundation, on which you can then build specialist skills and abilities. This gives you stability on which you can build performance. If we chase performance at the expense of stability we are trying to build a cannon on a canoe.

By building a broad base first you will then be far more likely to be able to achieve higher levels of performance while at the same time enjoying it more and staving off injury.

Anyone, regardless of age, ability, health status or injury should be able to work towards being fit for life. To be fit for life it's necessary to be competent in many domains of movement; join *all* of the following components of 'fitness' that will make your mind-body more robust.
- **Cardiovascular/respiratory endurance** – The ability to gather and use oxygen
- **Stamina** – The ability to use and store energy
- **Strength** – The ability of muscles to generate force
- **Flexibility** – The ability to maximise safe range of motion across joints

- **Power** – The ability of muscles to generate maximum force in minimum time
- **Speed** – The ability to do a repetitive movement in minimum time
- **Coordination** – The ability to combine multiple movements into one fluid movement
- **Agility** – The ability to change from one movement to another
- **Balance** – The ability to control your centre of gravity in relation to your support base
- **Accuracy** – The ability to control movement

Used with permission from Jim Crawley and Bruce Evans of Dynamax

Stable structure, able mind-body

Your mind-body can only activate these essential elements when you have stable structural alignment. Every bodily movement you do, whether swimming, deadlifts or yoga, depends on the integrity of your spine and the function of your nervous system. Subluxations of the spine will compromise the ability of your structure to bend, twist, lift, push, pull or any other movement. Subluxations also create nerve interference and distort the communication between brain and body so that your nervous system can't coordinate movements optimally.

With the structure compromised and the nervous system distorted with subluxations you'll be more prone to injury, slower to recover and you'll be sacrificing significant amounts of performance.

In our practice we work with competitive and professional athletes who want performance, as well as stay at home parents who want fitness and with children and babies whose parents want optimal development. The recipe for success is to always activate the fundamental first and then look to unleash performance. A stable structure is the most foundational thing in the pursuit of being fit for life and being able to Thrive!

As you're building your stable structure by correcting subluxations with a Chiropractor you can begin to address the essential elements and improve your competence in each.

Three types of movement to broaden the base

Your mind-body requires three categories of biologically appropriate movement in order to activate the growth and repair:

- MOVE MODERATELY
- MOVE HEAVY
- MOVE FAST

Adapted with permission from Mark Sisson

Move moderately

Move moderately every day

In the quest for biologically appropriate movement it's useful to start with the one you'll be doing most often. Moderate movement includes both the active things you might do for practise and play as well as the incidental types of movements you do all day like carrying shopping, climbing the stairs and even fidgeting. The latter of the two is called non-exercise activity thermogenesis, or NEAT, and is very important yet it gets little press.

Quit the sitting

By maximising the amount of movement we get in our everyday lives apart from dedicated play and practice, we can actually make a massive dent in the amount of defence and decay that modern living causes. Recently, popular studies have shown that sitting for hours at a time is very damaging to your health and raises your risk of cancer, heart disease, diabetes, obesity, depression and chronic pain. Australian research suggests that the average person spends only 73 minutes per day NOT sitting down. That's only 73 minutes for everything else including showering, cooking, shopping and exercising.

Sitting is damaging in two ways. The more you sit, the less you move and movement is a required nutrient that you are then deficient in. After sitting for one hour your fat burning enzymes go down by 90%. Secondly, because we sit in bad positions we tend to subluxate our spines. With a subluxation the structure of your body can't hold you up and you end up slumping. Slumping puts pressure on your nervous system and puts undue pressure on your heart and lungs as it closes down your chest. Subluxation creates dysfunction in how your brain gets information from your body and drives the defence and decay process even further causing more chronic inflammation. It also puts you at risk of injury when you do begin to move.

With so much sitting going on it's crucial to draw important distinctions. Studies show that if you're sitting all day then exercising for an hour a day you're still not undoing the damage that sitting causes. It seems like it's the lack of NEAT in our

219

day that is the major damaging factor. It's been found that by breaking up your sitting time with regular breaks you can prevent some of the effects caused by prolonged sitting. Those who take more regular breaks from a sitting position tend to have slimmer waistlines and better blood sugar balance.

Standing is an alternative to sitting that not only does less damage to your spinal structure but also encourages more NEAT. While you're standing it's easy to stand on one leg, swing one leg, bounce lightly and do all manner of small movements that help to activate your mind-body to growth and repair.

Quit the 'chronic cardio'

Wild free humans could move over long distances and do it very effectively. While they walked long distances daily, they didn't own a pair of trainers and set out on a tar road to accumulate mileage. One of our evolutionary advantages as hunters was that we could chase a springbok to exhaustion over the course of a day but we didn't do it at a constantly high pace and we didn't do it day in and day out.

With the popularity of jogging, triathlons, cycling, swimming and all other manner of endurance activities, not to mention every expert you've heard telling you that these things are good for you, it's going to seem a little odd that these might not be as good as you've been led to believe.

We've heard over and over how we can strengthen our heart and lungs as well as shed fat if we keep our heart rate up in the 'cardio zone' for as long as possible. In South Africa we have running and cycling built into our culture. It would seem odd not to see people on the road for some sort of race on a weekend, or a club doing a time trial during the week.

With the experts and our peers telling us to do more, here are some reasons to do less chronic, high-level training.

Joint damage

Driving along the road early on a Saturday morning and you're likely to see a stream of people participating in anything from a 5km to an ultra marathon (over 42km). Look at these people closely and you'll see their bodies don't look happy. The competitors will usually have limps, sloped shoulders, a head-chasing or hip-chasing running style, uneven gait, or they might just look plain uncomfortable.

These people will likely have subluxation of some sort that compromises their structure and their neurology system. Added to the damage the subluxations lead to on their own, this is where you get all those running injuries, from plantar fasciitis to stress fractures, from tendonitis to muscle strains and from osteoarthritis to back and neck pain. Each painful heal strike forces up to three times your body weight through the major joints in your body, and the damage accumulates, kilometre after kilometre.

Ask a group of long term runners about their injury history and you'll be astounded. This list will be long and detailed and they will all think it's normal. They have spent hours on physiotherapists' tables, hours in Chiropractor's offices, have had consults with surgeons and may have had a surprising number of joint replacements. The cost of endurance exercise on the structure of the body is very high.

Cycling is a very robotic movement that places abnormal stressors on the structure of the body because of the forced body position and the constricted, repetitive nature of the discipline. Besides only working the lower half of the body in a one dimensional and very artificial way, which can create structural imbalances, cycling is associated with lower bone density through the whole body, especially the lower back.

Chronic inflammation

By pushing your body to its limit for long periods of time on a regular basis you're forcing your body into defence and decay. While our body is capable of incredible endurance feats, it seems that doing this on tar roads and trails for hours at a time on a regular basis is not part of the plan. It has a very high metabolic cost.

When stressing your mind-body to the limit, whether on the road, in the gym or in an exam you're taxing the same stress response systems. Challenge your mind-body with a stress, whether physical, mental or chemical, and it responds by doing defence and you get oxidative stress. This is normal because we use the experience to get stronger if we are given time to recover. The problem arises when we accumulate mileage with little to no recovery time, because not only are we out pushing our body on the road a few days a week, we're also living stressful lives mentally as well as chemically through average nutrition.

This damage accumulates mile after mile, day after day and the stress and oxidative chemicals build up and do their damage, silently for the most part, for years before you realise how much damage you've done. When chronic inflammation rears its head it could be in the form of depression, heart disease or cancer or any other chronic, degenerative conditions we have covered.

Heart damage

The idea that doing endurance activities will strengthen your heart is a pervasive one. The problem is that there is very strong evidence to the contrary. The heart muscle is unlike any other. The muscle structure, its nerve supply and the way it uses nutrients are unique. When the heart is overworked, it doesn't tear like a hamstring or bicep, it gets enlarged and thickens. The heart is a hard worker and doesn't complain like your back or shoulder muscles might when they are tired. The heart quietly beats away and while we push our mind-body to the limit over and over it silently accumulates damage.

The result is that endurance athletes are at a significantly higher risk of abnormal electrical activities of the heart, called fibrillations, than non-runners, while moderate exercisers are at an even lower risk. Another study found, surprisingly, that marathon runners have more calcified plaque in the arteries to their heart.

What to do

The end goal here is to maximise your opportunities for movement and that means NEAT and dedicated play and practise time. Park in the space furthest from the shops and take a walk; walk or cycle instead of driving whenever possible; take the stairs instead of the lift or the escalators; walk to colleagues at work instead of emailing or phoning them. There are so many options for moving more, as soon as you start looking you'll find them.

For your dedicated play and practise movement it's useful to move for between 30 minutes to an hour a day at a moderate pace. A good guide here is that you should be out of breath but not so much that you can't hold a conversation. For the fitter amongst you that may be at 80-70% of your max heart rate and for others it will be at 50-60%.

STABILISE AND CORRECT – see a Chiropractor who knows how to assess your body for subluxations. If you are structurally compromised, work to stabilise and then correct your structure.

BROADEN THE BASE – gain competence in all of the foundational components of fitness listed above. If your base of physical competence is narrow, your foundation is weak. Not only will you be liable to injury but your performance will be significantly restricted. To broaden the base do all 3 types of biologically appropriate movements as described in this book. Move moderately, move heavy and move fast to build competence in all the elements of fitness.

VARIETY – Make sure you are varying the type of moderate movement you do, if not daily/weekly then do it seasonally. Variation in movement will keep your nervous system and structure challenged in a good way, forcing them to help you develop more competence in more domains of fitness. If you love running then swim, dance, row, skip or do anything else that moves you through different dimensions.

GET OUTSIDE – Be outside as much as you can. Sunshine is essential to our well-being and we get too little of it. Even if it's rainy, your mind-body has evolved to be water resistant too, so get out into the weather. Unlike wild humans, you can have a hot shower afterwards. Getting outside will also give you variation, whether it's navigating suburban streets, pavements and parks or getting out onto a trail. Get different surfaces under your feet whether grass, stones or bush and try to minimise the road and pavement.

PRACTICE RECOVERY – Give your mind-body time to recover from the stress of your practice while still being aware of the stress of your daily life. If you are doing a hard session then make sure you have a few light sessions in between; maximise your sleep, be the balance in your life and eat real food to grow and repair.

Taking all of this in context it's important to remember that "Why" and "How" you move are useful questions to ask first: what's your intent and what's your strategy?

If you love or are competitive in endurance activities you don't have to hang up your shoes or cleats right away. You can still continue your love affair with the road while minimising your risk of damage by observing the suggestions above.

Move heavy things

Moving heavy things is not only for people who want to build muscles; it's a biological requirement for health for every human being from children to the elderly. The benefits of lifting, pushing, pulling and pressing against resistance ranges from building lean body mass and generating strength, to preventing cardiovascular disease, diabetes, cancer, osteoporosis and back pain as well as promoting good blood lipid profiles and good blood pressure. All of these benefits can be gained in only 20 minutes twice a week. It also helps you to sleep better, improve your body image, sense of well-being and to look good naked!

Having all of these factors balanced is actually your normal state. Health and well-being is normal because your mind-body is innately intelligent. It is the deficiency of moving heavy things that predisposes us to illness and imbalance.

Safely stressing your structure, your nervous system, your cardiovascular system and your metabolism through lifting heavy things is vital to your ability to achieve vitality and Thrive! Your genes require the stimulation that heavy lifting gives and they trigger changes in your bones, joints, ligaments, muscles, heart, lungs, your nervous system, and your metabolism. Moving heavy things safely is a nutrient that switches on your growth and repair genes and switches off your defence and decay genes.

The goal behind moving heavy things is building strength to make you fit and strong enough to perform reasonably well at any physical task (like lifting the couch to clean, push-starting a car, getting up and down stairs, playing sports, lifting and carrying your kids) without causing discomfort or injury.

The by-product of strength training is being lean, having a good strength to weight ratio and being proportionately muscled. This is an useful component to looking good naked.

A universal principal for all people here, as in all parts of this book, is that you must move heavy things safely. Doing too much, and risking injury is just as counterproductive as doing too little. The more competent amongst us may be able to lift weights while others may have to start out learning how to move their own body weight again.

How much you move and how you move it, however, will depend on your state of health right now and your individual goals. What is very good for everyone to do is to observe the 3 'F's of move heavy.

Form

Form comes first because the quality of your movement matters more than how many repetitions you do or what weight you use. The biggest error we make when we move heavy is thinking that heavy is good, and heavier is better. The whole culture of the gym is built around that thought.

What might not be appreciated in the gym is that when you move heavy things the first thing you are stimulating is not the muscles, the bones or even the joints. The nervous system is the first thing you are stimulating. When you start a program of moving heavy things you might feel pretty weak but within 4-6 weeks you'll start to notice some improvement in your strength. By the 12 week mark you might even notice some more definition in a few muscles as well and the strength gains you've made.

This observation makes it tempting to think that you've been training muscles. The truth is it's your nervous system learning and adapting that has giving you those gains. Your brain and nerves have been learning how best to use your muscles, when to fire which one and when to rest another. This learning then sets into place patterns of movement that become ingrained in your brain – it's sometimes called 'muscle memory'.

It's a good idea to make sure you're creating good movement patterns, because bad ones lead to poor results and injury and are tough to change. Your brain can learn to dysfunction over time and it takes time to help it to unlearn poor habits. Crafting good movement patterns from now on will help you to make sure you are maximising results and minimising the risk of injuries.

Great form is the most effective means of achieving good results in the short and the long term. When you move properly you work the right things at the right time and get the best effect for your investment. A properly executed squat, for instance, will work your gluteal muscles more than it will your quadriceps.

Efficiency of your body movement leading to the best results for your practise and play time are best achieved when focussing on your form. By tapping into your body's natural movements you'll get better results in less time.

Functional

Next you can focus on what movements you are doing. The idea is to promote integration and balance in your mind-body to facilitate your growth and repair so you can experience vitality. For this to happen you need to move your mind-body in its natural, primal patterns. These patterns use synchronous groups and combinations of muscles, bones, joints, ligament and fascia. This goes against the common practise of isolating just one muscle group with one movement, like a bicep curl. Isolation leads to imbalance and dysfunction and the results of that are injury and an increasingly stuck and limited mind-body.

Functional movements are most efficient for getting the full range of physiological changes you are looking for. Epigenetic changes that drive hormone balance, immune strength, bone density, muscle strength and nervous system activation will happen best when we move functionally.

Using your innate movement patterns will get your nervous system firing much better and much faster. You will stimulate your brain and nerves while minimising stress on them. Benefits of this include memory, concentration, mood and focus.

Using functional movements you'll be activating and integrating the structure of your body that would normally be dysfunctional, inactive and imbalanced by isolated movements. The lesser known 'go' muscles for instance will be activated more than the 'show' muscle groups and this leads to better results for your training time. A more balanced physique will be the result, with less of the puffy weak muscles we see so much of. You'll also place less stress on your joints and help to keep them healthier for longer.

By moving your body the way it was meant to move, you'll also be making yourself more functional in daily life. Carrying kids and the shopping will be easier, carrying your school bag and your performance in sports will improve, push starting the car or changing a flat tyre will no longer terrify you and you'll be helping to injury-proof yourself in the process.

Full range of movement

Ideally you want to be aiming to work your joints through their full range of movement (ROM) whenever possible. You have to start somewhere, though, and it's a good thing to scale all your movements to your level of ability. If you can't do a push up you can do wall presses. If you can't do a full squat you can squat on a bench or against a wall. It's useful to work with a coach who can help you to identify your limitations and then work within them to start.

As you start to activate more mobility and experience more freedom in your movement you'll be sending more and more stimulation to your brain and getting more and more mind-body integration. That will drive better headspace as well as better physical results. This has the benefit of managing pain very well.

Working the structure of your body through its full range as much as possible will be a big boost to the effectiveness of your practise and play. As you get better and learn better patterns you'll feel stronger, more competent and more confident.

With the increased effective movement you'll notice more rapid changes. The efficiency of your time and energy spent moving heavy things will be greater than if you only moved yourself through limited ranges of motion. You'll be getting better results in less time.

Be the machine
The best way to get the most benefits will be to use your body in the way it was designed. That means avoiding machines unless there is a medical or other special need for them. Full body, full range of movement and functional movements are not what machines are for.

THE BASIC MOVES TO MASTER ARE:
- Animal walks
- Squats
- Lunges
- Deadlifts
- Kettlebell swings (Russian, not American)
- Bridges (Plank)
- Push-ups
- Pull-ups

The ideal
The principle we want to observe when moving heavy things is to use the minimum effective dose or MED – the smallest dose that will produce the desired result. Anything beyond MED is a waste. Think of MED like this: give a gift to a child on their birthday and their happiness levels will go up. Give them a second gift and

they go up some more but maybe not as much as they did for the first gift. As we give them more and more gifts the amount of happiness they feel will become less and less as each gift is added. Eventually you get to a point that another gift gives them no additional happiness and may begin to make them unhappy. If we used MED we would try to give them the smallest number of gifts that would produce the most happiness. Giving them more will only produce clutter and they won't play with them anyway.

Doing 10 repetitions of push ups might give you a certain benefit. Doing 20 repetitions does not necessarily give you twice the benefit; it might only be one and a half times the benefit. Doing 30 repetitions might only give 1.6 times the benefit of doing 10. So when we want the MED in this example we'll be doing about 10-15 reps.

Tim Ferriss, author of *The Four Hour Series,* is a big proponent of MED. One example he gives is doing kettle bell swings for 5 minutes 2-3 times a week.

Using MED means you will get the best rewards with the least effort and with the least risk of doing damage, because you're avoiding doing too much while at the same time getting great results. Looking around in many gyms, martial arts studios and CrossFit boxes, it becomes apparent that many people try to do too much too quickly and risk injury and over-training. Look at most people in a shopping mall and you'll notice that there are a lot of people doing too little. You want to find that sweet-spot.

MED will cover you for that and also take you a step further. Using this principle you can train smarter, not necessarily harder. Ideally it's useful to move heavy between 1-3 times a week, giving your mind-body adequate recovery time in between. We should be doing enough variation to keep our nervous system challenged and also enough regular programming to allow us to improve our movements.

Move fast

Very high intensity work over a short period of time is part of our genetic make-up and mimicking this movement creates very powerful changes in our bodies. An all out sprint in a short burst is an amazing thing. When you are pushing yourself as hard as you can you are feeding your mind-body nutrients and signalling your genes to activate growth and repair. Sprinting happens when you are moving at high intensities beyond the point where you use oxygen to get energy – the aerobic zone – and get into the anaerobic zone. You are essentially creating a short term 'state of emergency' in your body to reap the benefits.

The definition of sprinting is contingent on one important thing: safety. Pushing your mind-body further than it can tolerate and creating damage through over-training and injury is not useful; it's dangerous. Take time to get to know where your limitations are and proceed cautiously and with patience. If you keep an eye on MED and remain mindful of your form while sprinting you can do this safely and effectively. Recovery time is key to making sprinting effective, too.

Sprinting is a relative term. If you're exhausted after a walk around the block then sprinting will be a fast walk. If you're a seasoned runner then sprinting might be maximum effort hill runs. Be mindful of your form, as soon as the quality of your movement degrades then your sprint is done.

Your mind-body loves sprinting

Incorporating sprinting into your lifestyle in the form of intermittent bursts of movement followed by recovery can have some pretty amazing results. Use the short term stress response in your favour with this one. When you sprint it should consume all your faculties so you can't hold a conversation or wonder about your next car payment or school test. As you tax yourself physically it has a calming effect on the mind both while you're doing it and during the time afterwards.

Research confirms that an occasional burst of short, all- out physical effort can have a much more powerful effect on fitness – including endurance and especially on fat loss – than classic cardio, which takes much more time. One set of sprints (also known as 'high-intensity interval training' or HIIT) per week is all you need to improve speed, muscle mass, bone density, cardiovascular strength and aerobic capacity.

Sprints also affect your metabolic machinery by stimulating a surge of human growth hormone (HGH) and testosterone (beneficial for both men and women) and it can have an immune-boosting effect. HGH has been called the fountain of youth and the body's master craftsman and our levels decline over time, so that in your 40's they are a tenth of what they were during childhood. A sedentary lifestyle makes this decline even worse; the chemicals of defence and decay further clamp down on the hormone's release.

HGH is released when you get to the anaerobic threshold and the benefits include burning belly fat, building muscle fibres and boosting the volume of your brain. Some researchers see it as a way of reversing the modern signs of ageing including the loss of brain volume.

Compared to doing lower intensity movements, research shows that sprinting for as little as a thirty second burst will generate six times as much HGH. Another hormone boosted by sprinting is BDNF which you can think of as a fertiliser for your brain. Doing two sets of sprints can boost your BDNF levels significantly more than aerobic activities.

HIIT can improve your insulin sensitivity by twice as much as endurance training and improves your body's ability to burn fat. Your heart and blood vessels stay flexible and your lungs improve, too.

No other exercise modality gives as much reward for your effort. 15 to 20 minutes, from warm up to finish, and you're done. Before those of you who are out of shape, grossly overweight, older or have bad knees decide that this is not for you, you can definitely pursue low-impact options.

Sprinting can come in many forms and since we think of movement and not just exercise we can be much more creative with our activities. Essentially you'll be doing an intense movement at the highest speed you can safely do. So instead of just thinking about running, cycling, swimming and rowing you can add kids and dogs and make it a family affair. How about running in the pool or pushing and pulling a weighted sled? Do it on the beach, on a trail, in a forest or even in the corridor outside your bedroom. You can crawl, jump, climb, scurry, roll and a whole lot more.

You can use some movements from 'Move Heavy Things' and do them with lower weights and at an intense pace and still create a sprinting effect. This is an option used by gyms like CrossFit and can be very useful as long as we abide by the 3F's and MED.

High-Intensity Intermittent Training (HIIT)
With HIIT you will be working as hard as you safely can and then giving yourself time to recover. The recovery time is key; if you don't recover enough you can't push as hard in the next sprint and you don't get the benefits.

Tabata's are the classic HIIT routine used where you work hard for 20 seconds and then recover for 10 and repeat 8 times. In tests by Dr Tabata, trained cyclists using this protocol 4 times a week improved more than cyclists who were doing 60 minute training sessions 5 times a week. So in 32 minutes a week they did better than the other group doing 300 minutes week!

An issue with this is that the recovery time might be too short for most. If you can't recover enough between sprints then you can't really sprint and so you don't get the full benefit for your efforts. A protocol that overcomes this is a Gibala where you sprint for 30 seconds and recover for 4 minutes and repeat 4 times, giving more recovery time between sprints.

MED
When sprinting is done for too long and sessions are done without adequate recovery then we are taking the idea too far. Moving fast produces a short term stress response and if we do it too much it becomes a chronic stressor. Chronic stressors encourage the chemicals of defence and decay and the whole cascade of damage and degeneration they bring with them.

Spinning in gyms a few times a week is an example to doing too much. 'Fight Gone Bad' is a CrossFit workout that is a stretch too far for most people. Limiting Move Fast sessions to under 30 minutes, including workup and cool down, is a good guideline depending on how your mind-body handles it. If your sleep is disturbed, your energy drops or you can't perform mentally or physically the next day, then you're not recovering so reduce or remove sprinting for now and address sleep and recovery.

Go barefoot

When they were moving around, our ancestors would not have encountered endless miles of completely flat, hard surfaces like we do. They would have encountered grass, stones, rock, river sand, beach sand, pebbles and every other surface texture you can imagine. Their feet were strong and flexible and they used their built-in whole-body-shock-absorbing ability, mainly in the feet, legs and hips.

When we do move we're walking, running or jumping on completely flat, hard surfaces and hardly get any variation from that apart from when we might play sports on a grassy field. Even when we're doing that, though, we're in footwear that overly supports our supposedly fragile arches and they have cushioning in them that robs us of vital feedback we're supposed to get from our feet. Overly supportive, cushioned and rigid shoes create a deficiency in feedback and proprioception and can create structural misalignments. Our nervous system is at once robbed of feedback by the cushioning and also interfered with by the misalignments. That deactivates our shock absorbing system and causes our mind-body to structurally compensate leading to weakness, tightness, pain and predisposes us to injuries.

Athletic shoes as we know them are a very recent invention. In 1917 the first athletic shoes consisted of a thin rubber sole with a canvas top and no cushioning for the heel. Only in 1970 did Nike develop the running shoe with cushioned heels. This was a big backwards step for the mind-body as it stopped the foot moving naturally, which it had done for millions of years and robbed the brain of vital information about what was happening at the foot. Without this vital information the nervous system can't coordinate movement of the body appropriately and we begin to have the body break down.

As shoes have become more elaborate, more artificial and further confined our feet, our brain and bodies have weakened more and more. We've been putting our feet into compromising positions and then hammering our mind-body with a repetitive heel strike on tar for hours at a time and calling it healthy.

By getting more stimulation through your feet to your brain by going barefoot or by wearing minimalist shoes on natural surfaces you will strengthen and loosen your feet, strengthen and tone your legs and reactivate the muscles that become so dormant with our sitting lifestyles. Many types of pain and stiffness in the back, neck, legs and shoulders – not to mention headaches – respond very nicely to being closer to barefoot on natural surfaces.

Even being barefoot in the gym will make a massive difference. Try squatting, lunging or doing deadlifts barefoot instead of in shoes and notice the difference in your movement.

Running is best done barefoot or in minimalist shoes. If you're new to the idea then make sure you give yourself time to make the transition and work with a health care provider or coach who has experience with helping people transition. Err on the side of caution and take it slow.

Play hard, then rest

Life in the wild would have necessitated short bursts of high intensity work, like sprinting, fighting or climbing very quickly. This periodic high intensity exercise would have been followed by a prolonged period of rest and recovery. Your ancient biology expects such stimulus: sprint, recover, sprint, recover and without it you are deficient, defending and decaying.

Contrast this with the average pattern we see today. A few days a week we might do weights and cardio. Maybe we get our heart rate up on the treadmill or on the road for a few minutes, but not very regularly and usually not high enough.

HIIT is a fantastic way for us to mimic our natural movement pattern. Something to bear in mind here is that our ancestors had lots of down-time between sprinting episodes. High intensity days were followed by one or more low intensity days. This is important because high intensity work puts strain on your mind-body. Get enough recovery in between sessions and high intensity movement is a nutrient; not enough recovery and it's beginning to look like a toxin. If our rest is insufficient and we're sprinting or lifting too regularly we can create chronic inflammation that builds up and pushes us into defence and decay.

The same goes for regular long distance or endurance activities. Marathons, cycling, full distance triathlons, long distance paddling and other endurance activities can be healthy if done as part of a varied movement routine with adequate recovery. Chronic endurance activity creates chronic inflammation that leaches bones, cannibalises muscle and damages your heart.

A very good measure of your recovery from movement and life in general is your Heart Rate Variability (HRV). Recent technological advancements mean that there are smartphone apps that require no other special equipment to measure your HRV. These apps can then give you feedback and let you know how well you are resting and recovering.

A lower-tech way of assessing your recovery is by taking your heart rate first thing each morning before you get out of bed. Generally the lower it is the better rested you are. If your heart rate is raised then it's a sign your body is not fully recovered. The stressor that causes it could be mental (work stress, an upcoming assignment), chemical (stimulants affecting sleep) or physical (over-training). It could also be a sign that your body is fighting an infection and needs you to back off on the stressors for a few days.

Get outside
There is a body of thought that suggests that running on a treadmill doesn't mimic running the way it should. When you are running, you have to work to pull the road backwards so you can go forwards. On a treadmill that work is done for you and it disturbs your nervous system, can lead to structural imbalances, muscle weakness and injuries throughout spine, hips, legs, feet and ankles.

Wild free humans also moved outdoors; their environment did not include indoor gyms, tennis courts, pools or running tracks. They had access to sunshine and maintained great levels of vitamin D. When we try to mimic this with our movement we find that we enjoy ourselves much more, we connect to nature and are more likely to stick to a new movement program. Our indoor lifestyle is a massive departure from our genetic heritage

Move, rest, move
Rest was probably the most notable factor in the life of hunter-gatherers. As hard as they worked and played to get food and shelter they also enjoyed a lot of down time. This was not wasted time but gave their mind-bodies the space they need to recover after movement and repair, regenerate and restock their energy stores.

Professional athletes know this to be true. I've worked with many of them who are very protective over their down-time. It seems almost lazy to see them chilling out for hours on end but I've noticed that the ones who tend to keep themselves busy all day, even with small tasks, tend to be injured first.

Modern lifestyles are stressful and we have very little recovery time. We sleep less than ever, use more and more stimulants to keep us awake while at the same time sales of sleeping pills, tranquillisers and anti-anxiety medications are through the roof.

Find a tribe

For the sake of safety, especially when it involved hunting and gathering away from the settlement, wild free humans moved in tight knit social groups.

Hunting and gathering in groups just makes sense. Dancing, too, was an essential part of life, as part of rituals and celebrations for the whole tribe.

In most gyms you'll see people completely walled off from each other with their headphones in and staring at screens. They are isolated in the crowd. This seems like a massive move away from the connection our genes expect.

Team sports and sports clubs have fulfilled this role for us; they have connected us. The term 'comperation' describes how being part of a like minded community can help us with both cooperation and competition.

Recently group exercise methods have become very popular and in CrossFit, for instance, one of the things that keeps people coming back is the group environment where they feel they are part of a community and some even call it their tribe.

Once you start practising movement in a group it's much more fun, even if you're not a fan of team sports. When you make a commitment to another person to meet at a certain place and time and do a certain thing, you're more likely to follow through. Find a team or club that does what you enjoy, find a gym partner or join a community. ●

Those who do not move do not notice their chains.
ROSA LUXEMBURG

13

Rest & restore

Your star-gazing physiology.
Idleness is productive.

Sleep

Creatures of habit

The ecosystem that is your mind-body is always in a delicate dance between what happens on the outside and what happens on the inside, between you and your environment. We have learned that our genes respond to our environment in a sort of dance. Factors in our environment like our movement and our nutrition are signals that our genes respond like a dancer moving to a beat.

All of the cycles and rhythms that happen in nature affect us in powerful and profound ways. These cycles influence our physiology and can help us move towards growth, repair and vitality.

Through our evolution over millions of years the most consistent and powerful environmental signal that has moulded our genes is the cycle of day and night, light and dark. The most primitive of single-celled life forms we study today change their physiology in response to sunlight. As we've developed through eons into complex multicellular life, the sun and the light it provides everyday followed by darkness every night is constant.

As the seasons change so does the length of day and night and the amount of light and dark our ancient biology has experienced. This force is so strong in living things that it causes trees to shed their leaves, makes some animals slow their metabolism to a near death like state of hibernation and makes others migrate thousands of kilometres across the globe.

These natural rhythms form a delicate waltz between our mind-body and the motion of our planet that affect our physiology. When we're in tune with them we're creating growth and repair for vitality and when we are out of tune we are creating defence and decay for lost human potential and disease.

Day and night, summer and winter – these are rhythms and cycles we have been exposed to since the dawn of life and they have fundamentally affected our evolution. We have inherited an ancient physiology that is a celestial clock-watcher. We call our response to these natural cycles our circadian rhythm.

Even when our early hominid ancestors began using fire about 800 000 years ago studies suggest that early man still went to bed after the sun went down and got up just before the dawn. It was with the advent and spread of electric lighting in the twentieth century that humanity created near perpetual daylight and disrupted that most basic cycle our physiology craves.

"Sleep when you're dead!" is a modern creed that industrialised culture lives by. More and more sleep is seen as something to be put off in our lives lived in busyness. As animals that are at odds with nature's laws, when we negate one of our most basic drives – to periodically rest and restore – we pay the price.

Being out of sync with daily cycles triggers the defence pathways we've explored, leading to chronic inflammation as part of a state of decay and to chronic disease. If you're unable to lose weight or gain muscle, if you're struggling with fatigue or focus during the day, if you have on-going aches, pains and muscle tightness or if you're just underperforming and not being as productive as you want to be your sleeping may be the issue.

It's not just how much you sleep that matters, your quality of sleep is also important. Poor sleeping patterns are strongly associated with cancer, heart disease, depression, obesity, diabetes, chronic pain, anxiety, learning disorders, frequent injuries, PCOS and much more.

Sleep is a nutrient

Sleep is a physiological process that has interested and confounded researchers. While we have learned a lot about sleep there is still a lot we don't know. It used to be thought that sleep was a passive state where your brain and body 'turned off' to rest from our daily activities. Now we know that your brain can be even more active while you are sleeping than when you are awake.

In very simple terms sleep is an active process for our mind-body to rest and restore. The cellular structure of the brain changes when you sleep, the spaces between cells get bigger. This allows the brain to flush out toxic molecules associated with brain degeneration that build up in those spaces. When we're asleep our mind-body produces melatonin, one of our most powerful antioxidants. This hormone is more effective at suppressing some cancers than any drug we know of. It has a potent effect on the immune system, and counters that infamous trouble-maker – chronic inflammation – and helps us to 'deflame'.

While we're going through healthy sleep cycles our immune system tends to the garden that is our microbiome, trimming away the colonies of bacteria, viruses, yeast, fungi and parasites that live within us. Our microbiome is immensely important to our well-being but if it becomes overgrown we will grow ill. In fact some theories suggest that this immune activity in response to our gut flora that makes us tired and is a powerful trigger for sleep. This would seem to make some sense of why you want to sleep so much when you have a cold or flu.

While you sleep your brain is preparing for the next day, growing new neural connections, consolidating memories and sorting through all the information that came at you during the day. This is healthy sleep. The term beauty sleep is not far off the truth: your cells and organs use sleep to grow and repair and resist the effects of stressors that cause ageing. From gut and skin to your heart, lungs and blood vessels, they all do the majority of their repairs and maintenance while you are in slumber.

The balance of hormones like insulin, leptin, growth hormone and many others is dependent on healthy sleep. Our reproductive cycles hinge on healthy sleep and without it they become deranged. Imbalanced hormones mean poor growth and development, accelerated ageing with faster physical and mental decline, low libido, fertility and reproductive issues. It means you won't be able to lose fat and getting strong will be near impossible.

With all of this it's easy see why sleep is a vital nutrient and how poor sleep can be a deficiency that leads to defence and decay, leads to a smaller life and disease too.

How do we sleep?

When someone overindulges in alcohol and goes into what seems like a deep sleep their brain waves go into a state that is almost coma-like. When the person wakes up they don't feel rested and they feel like they need more sleep, even though they may have 'slept' for more than 9 hours, but in fact passed out.

Restful sleep happens when your brain cycles between lighter rapid eye movement (REM) sleep and deeper non-REM phases. Through the night you cycle between NREM and REM phases.

The overindulging person doesn't cycle as well between these phases of sleep and so doesn't feel rested in the morning. Chemicals that have a stimulating effect (like caffeine) or a depressant effect (like alcohol or sleeping pills) interfere with your sleep cycles and therefore your rest and recovery.

Our most powerful trigger for sleep is darkness. As the sun goes down it brings darkness and that triggers the release of melatonin to help us sleep. During the night we go through our sleep phases and melatonin levels then drop away in the early hours of the morning, as the sun begins to rise, helping us wake up fully rested, ready for a new day.

Effects of limiting sleep

We know that light in your eyes can disturb your sleep cycles, but in 1998 two researchers from Cornell University got 15 people into a sleep lab and ran some tests on them. What they found was surprising. By shining a blue light behind their subject's knees they managed to disturb sleep cycles and melatonin release. This suggests that it's not just the light your eyes pick but all light in your environment that affects your circadian rhythm!

The brighter the light the more it affects you and blue/white light affects you more than orange/red light. Think fluorescent light versus campfire light. The screens of TV's computers, phones and tablets are all deeply stimulating and are a strong signal to your mind-body to wake up and stay awake.

Without sufficient quality and quantity of sleep your mind-body won't be able to effectively repair the damage that living creates. We live in a time of extreme daily stressors and our mind-body needs all the recovery it can get. The result of chronic poor sleep is a state of defence creating chronic inflammation during a time when your mind-body is supposed to be quelling inflammation. Our stress chemicals like cortisol go way up instead of down. Chronic inflammation is the chemical cocktail of defence turning to decay. We've explored how it is linked to almost every chronic disease from heart disease to cancer. Now when you are not sleeping well you not only don't get to 'deflame' but you also generate more inflammation. Chronic inflammation along with the reduced immune activity that a lack of sleep quality and quantity brings sets you up for infections, allergies and autoimmune issues.

The link between cancer and poor sleep is strong in research, so strong in fact, that in 2009 Denmark paid compensation to women who worked night shifts for their increased risk of developing cancer. Hormone imbalances, chronic inflammation and sleep disturbance go hand in hand; it is a state of defence and decay. Insulin and leptin are hormones that affect how much fat you carry. Your sensitivity to these hormones and your ability to tolerate carbohydrates and shed fat is very much a sleep and inflammation driven phenomena.

If you're using nutrition and movement to manage your weight and you're not getting enough good sleep then you might be undermining all your efforts. One of the best pieces of advice those who want to rid themselves of excess fat can get is to get enough quality sleep. Just one night of 4 hours of sleep will affect how your body handles insulin and 6,5 hours instead of 8 hours is enough to cause men's fat metabolism to fall by two thirds.

Exposure to light in your room or from your screen delays your melatonin release. You don't sleep as well and you're not as sharp as you could be the next morning. It's another form of stimulant, like caffeine, that can have a toxic affect on your physiology. A change in how you produce and use melatonin will have powerful affects on how well you function. Instead of just making you a little groggy the next day, chronic issues can result. Dysfunction in melatonin physiology has been linked to the ADHD spectrum of issues.

How to get good quality sleep

Parenting a toddler teaches you a lot about life. One big lesson is that little people often can't go from awake to asleep straight away. They need to be calmed and prepared for sleep, it helps to have a routine to help them get themselves into a state of sleepiness. Any parent who has been frustrated by their child's lack of cooperation around bedtime knows what I mean.

Your mind-body operates much like a toddler's. Even if you're fatigued at the end of the day, it's very useful to give yourself cues that it's time to go from awake to asleep. Anchoring the transition from arousal to sleepiness on rituals and habits makes it more likely that you will have better sleep patterns and reap the rewards. These cues as well as a list of things not to do I call 'sleep hygiene'.

Sleep hygiene

Use this list to create routines. Start somewhere and then build on it, don't try to do all of them at once.

PHYSICAL
- Try to get sensible sun exposure during the day, preferably in the morning.

242

This helps to set your day/nights cycles on the right path early in the day.
- Dim the lights at least an hour before bed; go for soft orange and red light that mimics firelight. Candles are great.
- Avoid all screens for at least an hour before. Their stimulating effect is potent and can affect not just how quickly you can fall asleep but also your sleep cycles. Even background TV can be a distraction that gives your mind-body the signal to stay awake.
- Create complete electrical darkness in your bedroom. Exclude all electrical light from things like streetlights and house lights; blackout curtains or blinds are a good idea. Cover all lights, even if they are small indicator lights on appliances. If you can't see your hand in front of your face you're doing well!
- Make sure your room is a little cooler than the rest of your house. Your body temperature needs to fall slightly to get into your sleep cycles and if you're too hot it can inhibit good sleep.
- Keep as close to a routine as possible, even on the weekends. I've noticed that going down and waking up at roughly the same time everyday helps to set your physiology up for good sleep cycles.

CHEMICAL
- Avoid stimulants like caffeine and nicotine for 7 hours before bed. The effects of that coffee at lunch can last for a lot longer than you realise. Even if you don't feel hyped up on caffeine and fall asleep well enough, it could still affect your sleep cycles. Green tea has more than just caffeine, theophylline is also a potent stimulant.
- Avoid depressants like alcohol, and medication if possible for at least 4 hours before bed. Painkillers, anti-inflammatories and antihistamines are classic examples to be avoided if possible. A glass of wine at night may help you to chemically unwind but it's going to rob you of some good quality sleep cycles.
- Minimise your sugar and starch intake. Chronic overconsumption of sugary and starchy foods breeds hormone disruption and that will affect your mind/body's ability to enter into restful sleep.

MENTAL
- Stay away from social media and your email for an hour before bed. These are strongly stimulating and there is very little happening in the world that can't wait until the next day.

- Read a fiction book. A real paper book if at all possible. Fiction engages your imagination and helps you to disengage from the day and any stressors that might have occurred. Sit and read to your kids or quietly with your partner and making bonding time too.
- Some form of mindfulness or meditation in the evenings is useful to allow your mind-body to process some of the accumulated information that it has absorbed.
- Talk through your day with a friend, partner or children. It helps you to process the events of the day and calm your mind. We've done this with our daughter since she was born and we notice that when we do it for her and ourselves we all have much better sleep.

How much is enough?

You know you are getting enough sleep when you wake up feeling refreshed without an alarm clock. If you're not there yet, then you know you need better sleep and you need more of it.

Sharpen the axe

> *Give me six hours to chop down a tree*
> *and I will spend the first four sharpening the axe.*
> ABRAHAM LINCOLN

Downtime = productive time

There is a very specific feeling I get when I know that it's time. When I start hopping from one task to another without finishing any of them, I know it's time. When I find it tough to make a decision, even what to have for lunch, I know it's time. When I feel this starting I say that my mind is 'losing traction' and the 'wheels are starting to spin.'

This feeling tells me two things. I probably didn't prepare my mind-body well enough at the start of the day and taking a step back from my tasks and doing nothing for a while would best serve me. I might take out my juggling balls, do some gentle movements or sit and meditate to help my mind-body decompress, filter and integrate.

I pay special attention to that urge to 'just get back to work' and realise that this is not the right thing to do right now. When this feeling goes on for a few days I know I should have taken a holiday a week ago.

Modern consumerism and a drive for achievement to fill the holes in our soul drive us to be ever busier and to 'get more done'. The chronic message is that we need to work harder and do more.

In that mindset, sitting quietly for some time each day does not seem like a productive thing to do, it might even seem like a waste of time. Taking a holiday is what other people get to do but not you, you're too busy.

The late Stephen Covey the author, educator and businessman called it Sharpening the Saw and made it his 7th Habit in the international bestselling book the *7 Habits Of Highly Effective People*.

"Idleness is not just a vacation, an indulgence or a vice; it is as indispensable to the brain as vitamin D is to the body, and deprived of it we suffer a mental affliction as disfiguring as rickets," writes essayist Tim Kreider in The New York Times. "The space and quiet that idleness provides is a necessary condition for standing back from life and seeing it whole, for making unexpected connections and waiting for the wild summer lightning strikes of inspiration – it is, paradoxically, necessary to getting any work done."

On all levels, mentally, emotionally, physically, metabolically and even spiritually we are well served by creating downtime on a regular basis. When we do this and allow our min/body and spirit to rest, restore and recharge we can return to the world of 'getting thins done' with a renewed sense of fun and a bigger impact.

Slow down to go faster
In my practice I use the 5 minutes a day principle to get people started and those who do it notice some difference within a few days. Most like it so much they progress onto 10 to 40 minutes a day. They feel like they are getting more done and feeling less stressed.

There is no one who can't make 5 minutes a day, find a quiet spot and do a gentle focus exercise. One person I worked with sat under their desk in their open plan office and listened to some soothing music for their 5 minutes during the week.

You might observe your breath, counting 5 seconds inhale and 5 seconds exhale for 5 minutes. When you mind wonders, let the focus gently return to your breath.

Like the person who hid under the desk, maybe music is your calming tonic and for some it's a picture or some form of visualisation. The point is that there are lots of ways to use your 5 minutes, all you need it 5 minutes.

After reading this far into the book you might realise that combining it with your 5 minutes a day movement is a good idea and now you're multiplying the effect on your life.

Taking a few moments out of the busy-ness of the lives we've created for ourselves will help us get more from the time, energy and attention allotted to us and make a bigger impact in the world.

Go away to come back
Learning French made me a better doctor. I was going to be in rural France in a small village where only one person spoke any English so I had no choice really, I had to learn some French. I didn't take it too seriously; this was going to be a holiday after all so I learned the greetings and a few other phrases to see me through.

The first week I felt like I understood nothing except hello and goodbye. I could introduce myself but then couldn't understand anything they said back to me. By the second week I was getting a few words here and there and by week three I was able to follow a conversation even thought I couldn't really add to it.

The effect of being in a new place, learning a new language and doing new things was amazing. My inspiration in practice that had begun to wane came flooding back. I was having ideas about how better to serve the people I was seeing and ways we could improve the practice. I was making new connections and possibilities where before I was only feeling frustration.

Getting your mind-body into new situations and surroundings has a magical effect. Learning a new sport, a new language or taking up a new hobby is a great way to keep your mind-body young. By engaging in new and novel things you keep your brain and body active, learning and engaged. Try to do something in a new physical location too and if you can immerse yourself in these activities for days to weeks at a time by travelling or going to a seminar, you can get maximum value for your efforts.

Here are some ideas to get you started:
- Schedule time out of your daily routine at least once a week to go somewhere or do something new. A new park, beach, walking/running/cycling route, restaurant, museum. Go rock climbing, go-karting, making pottery, gardening, sing karaoke, learn a new movement or sport or enrol in a course – the more foreign it is to you, the better.
- Schedule holidays and go somewhere you've never been. Go camping if you're used to hotels, head to the mountains if you're used to the beach go to a farm if you're used to the city. Take on a new culture or language with new food and new customs. Learn their history and listen to their stories.

None of these suggestions needs to cost much money. You would be surprised at what is available in and around your home when you begin looking.

To live a bigger life it is very useful to be powerfully present. Present at home, present and work and present when doing the things we love most. Resting and restoring by sharpening the axe and going away to come back are effective and efficient ways to maximise your personal potential. You ability to live, love, work, play, serve, experience and create. ●

> *Creation is a better means of self-expression than possession;*
> *it is through creating, not possessing, that life is revealed.*
> VIDA D. SCUDDER

CONCLUSION

THE PURPOSE OF THIS BOOK is to help you to live a bigger life by proactively investing in your well-being. We all live busy lives: the demands on our time, energy and attention are constantly being pulled in many different directions at once. In the midst of this there is a way to dance through the chaos of life. It is not a quick fix, though you can see results soon.

It is a challenging path to walk but it can also be easier than you think. It can feel lonely until you meet more souls like you who are looking for more than immediate gratification; there are many of us. A vitalistic lifestyle is one that promotes your mindful awareness, helps you move toward vitality and helps you consciously create the life you dream of by discovering new possibilities and activating your mind-body's ability to Thrive!

We have taken a journey through your values, your beliefs and through many aspects of your lifestyle. We started the first section with our society's beliefs around health and how they might be harming us. The second section delved into the principles that underlie a vitalistic lifestyle and the last section looked at how we might implement theses principles: eating, moving, thinking, sleeping, nature and breathing were all addressed. We also looked at Chiropractic in a new light though it has been practised for over 100 years.

"Hope is a good thing, maybe the best of things and no good thing ever dies." (*Rita Hayworth and The Shawshank Redemption* by Stephen King)

You have the ability to do more, love more, serve more, experience more and create more than you think you can. To get to a different result in our lives we have to be prepared to do new things and the prerequisite for doing anything new in life is hope. Hope that things could be better. It is my hope that some of the ideas in this book feed your sense of hope and help you to take action steps to improve your experience of life.

New discoveries seem to come ever faster and over the 3 years of writing this book the progress of science has caused me to update my work on a number of occasions and even change my mind on a few matters. As new evidence emerges some details in this book will become outdated. What won't change are the principles of biology that we have explored together. Remember that we are intelligent ecosystems within larger ecosystems and we use this premise to ask new questions to make new discoveries.

There is one more thing that is useful for you to bear in mind: everything in this book could be wrong.

Dr Greg Venning
Cape Town
April 2016

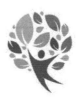

ACKNOWLEDGEMENTS

MY FIRST and biggest thank you goes to Eils, my wife: it feels like we wrote this together. You have taught me so much about living a better life and have held my hand as I wrote each word. Both you and Breah have been so patient while this has been created and for putting up with my manic writing process. I promise I'll take a break before starting number two!

The main ideas in the book are not my own, they have been around for centuries. I have had the privilege to stand on the shoulders of those who have come before me and I hope I have been able to add something useful to our conscious evolution. Dr Mark Postles, you have been a way-shower on my journey from our first meeting and your elegantly powerful and probing questions always facilitate deeper understanding and more effective action in all areas of my life.

For your great teaching and ethical compass with your vision and execution of a new paradigm of real healthcare, Dr James Chesnut, thank you; with your insightful urging Dr Patrick Gentempo, you pushed me to see the bigger picture and realise the power of clarifying my philosophy; Dr Simon Floreani and Dr Jennifer Bonham-Floreani – you are a constant reminder of how a life lived with intention can change the world, be fun and attract prosperity.

An unexpected inspiration I met on a chance trip to The Netherlands was Dr Vismai Schonfelder who has been a member of my mental board of directors ever since; Dr John Demartini's teaching on life has guided me through many decisions and enriches my existence.

It is a blessing to be in the Chiropractic profession and to be surrounded by so many smart, hard working and fun-loving individuals who serve humanity in their lives everyday. A special mention to Drs Martin Cook, Adam Smith, Matthew Doyle, Hayden Belle, Jaime Pinillos, Julie Reynolds, Megan Clubb, Jonothan Evans, Robert Delgado, Travis Mitchell, Adam Sayers, Brett Lederlie and Jason Fyfer. You guys know me inside out and for whatever reason are still my friends, thank you!

To each person who I have been blessed enough to serve as a sports coach, Chiropractor, transformative coach and speaker I am deeply grateful. Each time I teach, adjust, coach or speak I learn more about myself and gain a deeper understanding of the ideas I present.

To quote my grandfather, "The privileged education afforded me in my youth instilled in me a deep sense of duty." King Edward VII High School was a significant learning ground and formed a large part of my young life. The University of Johannesburg grounded me in basic science and gave me many opportunities to take leadership roles that helped me discover my values. There was an inflection point in my life without which my path would have been very different: The World Congress of Chiropractic Students (WCCS) held in Denmark in 2005 exposed me to remarkable people and new ideas. Over the years the people involved in WCCS have tested my paradigm and led me down exciting new paths of discovery and experience and become fantastic friends.

Despite what the cover says, a book is never the work of just the people listed as the authors. The team behind those names is vitally important. My editor, Robin Stuart-Clark, was a critical factor in bringing this project. The work of Robin's team at Publishing Print Matters and his support and constructive criticism has been immense.

Good friends challenge you as much as they support you. Alan Golding taught me how to question my own assumptions and dared me to do more; Bryan Banfield teaches me about living a life of significance and Rika Geyser is the ultimate way shower for living your life authentically.

Last but definitely not least I thank my family: how do you show genuine gratitude to your family for their role in your life? They are there from the beginning and help you in so many ways that you are never aware of. To my parents, William and Julie Venning, you gave me everything, you are endlessly nurturing, you ask me the hard questions when needed and you support my decisions with love. I am the youngest of three and my siblings always looked out for me. Andrew you have always been someone that lights the path ahead of me and Nicky you are a trusted confidant, advisor and friend. However life happens I am so grateful that you are my family.

BIBLIOGRAPHY

Abdulla, Jawdat, and Jens Rokkedal Nielsen. "Is the risk of atrial fibrillation higher in athletes than in the general population? A systematic review and meta-analysis.." *Europace : European pacing, arrhythmias, and cardiac electrophysiology : journal of the working groups on cardiac pacing, arrhythmias, and cardiac cellular electrophysiology of the European Society of Cardiology* 11.9 (2009): 1156–1159.

Action to Control Cardiovascular Risk in Diabetes Study Group et al. "Effects of intensive glucose lowering in type 2 diabetes.." *New England Journal of Medicine* 358.24 (2008): 2545–2559.

Ahlbom, A et al. "Cancer in twins: genetic and nongenetic familial risk factors.." *Journal of the National Cancer Institute* 89.4 (1997): 287–293.

Alegria-Torres, Jorge Alejandro, Andrea Baccarelli, and Valentina Bollati. "Epigenetics and lifestyle.." *Epigenomics* 3.3 (2011): 267–277.

Aspden, Phillip, ed. *Preventing Medical Errors.* Washinton DC: Institute of Medicine: Committee on Identifying and Preventing Medication Errors, 2007.

Bakris, G et al. "Atlas vertebra realignment and achievement of arterial pressure goal in hypertensive patients: a pilot study.." *Journal of human hypertension* 21.5 (2007): 347–352.

Barham-Floreani, J, and S Floreani. *The Legitimacy of Chiropractic in Family Health care.* Well Adjusted, September 3, 2013.

Bernstein, Lenny. "Fit at 102." *Washington Post*, n.d. Online. Internet. 17 Jan. 2016. Available: https://www.washingtonpost.com/local/fit-at-102/2013/03/12/786a7e96-8346-11e2-b99e-6baf4ebe42df_story.html.

Bjelakovic, Goran, Dimitrinka Nikolova, Lise Lotte Gluud, Rosa G Simonetti, and Christian Gluud, 'Mortality in Randomized Trials of Antioxidant Supplements for Primary and Secondary Prevention', Journal of the American Medical Association, 297 (2007), 842

Bjelakovic, Goran et al. "Mortality in Randomized Trials of Antioxidant Supplements for Primary and Secondary Prevention." *JAMA* 297.8 (2007): 842.

Bloom, D E, E T Cafiero, E Jan e Llopis, S Abrahams-Gessel, L R Bloom, S Fathima, A B Feigl, T Gaziano, M Mowafi, A Pandya, K Prettner, L Rosenberg, B Seligman, A Z Stein, and C Weinstein. "The Global Economic Burden of Non-communicable Diseases." *World Economic Forum* (2012): 1–48.

Boden, William E et al. "Impact of Optimal Medical Therapy With or Without
    Percutaneous Coronoary Intervention on Lont-Term Cardiovascular End
    Points in Patients With Stable Coronary Artery Disease (from the Courage
    Trial." *The American Journal of Cardiology* 104.1 (2009): 1–4.

Booth, Frank W et al. "Waging war on physical inactivity: using modern
    molecular ammunition against an ancient enemy.." *Journal of applied
    physiology (Bethesda, Md. : 1985)* 93.1 (2002): 3–30.

Breig, A. *Biomechanics of the Nervous System: Breig revisited.* Ed. M Shacklock.
    First. Adelaide: Neurodynamic Solutions, 2007.

Brickman, P, Brickman, P, D Coates, D Coates, R Janoff-Bulman, and R Janoff-
    Bulman, 'Lottery Winners and Accident Victims: Is Happiness Relative?',
    Journal of Personality and Social Psychology, 36 (1978), 917–27

Brickman, P et al. "Lottery winners and accident victims: is happiness relative?."
    Journal of personality and social psychology 36.8 (1978): 917–927.

Cailliet, René, and Leonard Gross. "The rejuvenation strategy" (1988).

Campbell, S S, and P J Murphy. "Extraocular Circadian Phototransduction
    in Humans." *Science* 279.5349 (1998): 396–399. Available: http://www.
    sciencemag.org/cgi/doi/10.1126/science.279.5349.396.

Carney, Dana R, Amy J C Cuddy, and Andy J Yap. "Power Posing: Brief Nonverbal
    Displays Affect Neuroendocrine Levels and Risk Tolerance." *Psychological
    Science* 21.10 (2010): 1363–1368.

Chen, E et al. "Genome-wide transcriptional profiling linked to social class in
    asthma." *Thorax* 64.1 (2009): 38–43.

Chestnut, J. *Innate Physical Fitness & Spinal Hygiene.* Victoria: The Wellness
    Practice, 2005.

Chottanapund, Suthat et al. "Anti-aromatase effect of resveratrol and melatonin
    on hormonal positive breast cancer cells co-cultured with breast adipose
    fibroblasts.." *Toxicology in vitro : an international journal published in
    association with BIBRA* 28.7 (2014): 1215–1221.

Citation: Kandel, E R, J H Schwartz, T M Jessell, S A Siegelbaum, and A J
    Hudspeth, Principles of Neural Science. Fourth Edition. McGraw-Hill. 2000.,
    Fifth Edition (McGraw-Hill, 2012)

Cole, S W et al. "Accelerated course of human immunodeficiency virus infection
    in gay men who conceal their homosexual identity.." *Psychosomatic medicine*
    58.3 (1996): 219–231.

Cole, S W et al. "Elevated physical health risk among gay men who conceal their
    homosexual identity.." *Health psychology : official journal of the Division of*

Health Psychology, American Psychological Association 15.4 (1996): 243–251.

Cole, S W, M E Kemeny, and S E Taylor. "Social identity and physical health: accelerated HIV progression in rejection-sensitive gay men.." *Journal of personality and social psychology* 72.2 (1997): 320–335.

Dobbs, David. "The Social Life of Genes." *psmag.com*, n.d. Online. Internet. 18 Nov. 2015. Available: http://www.psmag.com/books-and-culture/the-social-life-of-genes-64616.

Donga, Esther et al. "A single night of partial sleep deprivation induces insulin resistance in multiple metabolic pathways in healthy subjects.." *The Journal of clinical endocrinology and metabolism* 95.6 (2010): 2963–2968.

Doyle, Matthew F. "Is chiropractic paediatric care safe? A best evidence topic." *Clinical Chiropractic* 14.3 (n.d.): 97–105.

Duvivier, Bernard M F M et al. "Minimal intensity physical activity (standing and walking) of longer duration improves insulin action and plasma lipids more than shorter periods of moderate to vigorous exercise (cycling) in sedentary subjects when energy expenditure is comparable.." *PloS one* 8.2 (2013): e55542.

Edwards, Ian J, Susan A Deuchars, and Jim Deuchars. "The intermedius nucleus of the medulla: a potential site for the integration of cervical information and the generation of autonomic responses." *Journal of chemical neuroanatomy* 38.3 (2009): 166–175.

Ekblom-Bak, Elin et al. "The importance of non-exercise physical activity for cardiovascular health and longevity." *British Journal of Sports Medicine* 48.3 (2014): 233–238.

Fallon, Joan. "The effect of chiropractic treatment on pregnancy and labor: a comprehensive study." *Proceedings of the World Federation of Chiropractic* (1991): 24–31.

Forencich, F. *Change Your Body, Change The World.* Exuberant Animal Books, 2010.

Fredericson, Michael, and Anuruddh K Misra. "Epidemiology and aetiology of marathon running injuries.." *Sports medicine (Auckland, N.Z.)* 37.4-5 (2007): 437–439.

Gibala, Martin J et al. "Physiological adaptations to low-volume, high-intensity interval training in health and disease." *The Journal of Physiology* 590.5 (2012): 1077–1084.

Goren-Inbar, Naama et al. "Evidence of hominin control of fire at Gesher Benot Ya'aqov, Israel.." *Science* 304.5671 (2004): 725–727.

Gottlieb, M S. "Neglected spinal cord, brain stem and musculoskeletal injuries stemming from birth trauma.." *Journal of Manipulative and Physiological Therapeutics* 16.8 (1993): 537–543.

Grant, William B. "The Geographic Variation in the Prevalence of Attention-Deficit/Hyperactivity Disorder in the United States Is Likely Due to Geographic Variations of Solar Ultraviolet B Doses and Race." *Biological Psychiatry* 75.3 (2014): e1.

Great Britain, Fitness Industry Association. "Winning the Retention Battle: Reviewing Key Issues of UK Health & Fitness Club Membership Retention" (2001).

Gurven, M, and H Kaplan. "Longevity among hunter-gatherers: a cross-cultural examination." *Population and Development Review* (2007).

Haavik, Heidi, and Bernadette Murphy. "Subclinical Neck Pain and the Effects of Cervical Manipulation on Elbow Joint Position Sense." *Journal of Manipulative and Physiological Therapeutics* 34.2 (2011): 88–97.

Haavik, Heidi, and Bernadette Murphy. "The role of spinal manipulation in addressing disordered sensorimotor integration and altered motor control.." *Journal of electromyography and kinesiology : official journal of the International Society of Electrophysiological Kinesiology* 22.5 (2012): 768–776.

Hamilton, Marc T, Deborah G Hamilton, and Theodore W Zderic, 'Role of Low Energy Expenditure and Sitting in Obesity, Metabolic Syndrome, Type 2 Diabetes, and Cardiovascular Disease.', Diabetes, 56 (2007), 2655–67 <http://dx.doi.org/10.2337/db07-0882>

Heron, Melonie. "Deaths: leading causes for 2008.." *National Vital Statistics Report* 60.6 (2012): 1–94.

Jackson, T, and A Harper. "Blunders will never cease. How the media report medical errors. A risky business." *BMJ* 322.7285 (2001): 562.

Kado, Deborah M et al. "Hyperkyphotic Posture and Poor Physical Functional Ability in Older Community-Dwelling Men and Women: The Rancho Bernardo Study." *The journals of gerontology. Series A, Biological sciences and medical sciences* 60.5 (2005): 633–637.

Karsenty, Gerard. "The complexities of skeletal biology.." *Nature* 423.6937 (2003): 316–318.

Kaufman, Joan et al. "Social supports and serotonin transporter gene moderate depression in maltreated children.." *Proceedings of the National Academy of Sciences of the United States of America* 101.49 (2004): 17316–17321.

Kilo, Charles M, and Eric B Larson. "Exploring the harmful effects of health care.." *JAMA* 302.1 (2009): 89–91.

Kirsch, Irving. "Antidepressants and the Placebo Effect." *Zeitschrift für Psychologie* 222.3 (2014): 128–134.

Kreider, Tim. "The 'Busy' Trap." *New York Times*, n.d. Online. Internet. 30 Jun. 2012. Available: http://opinionator.blogs.nytimes.com/2012/06/30/the-busy-trap/?_r=0.

Lancaster, H O. "Expectations of Life: A Study in the Demography, Statistics, and History of World Mortality." *Springer Science & Business Media* (1990).

Lennon, John et al. "Postural and respiratory modulation of autonomic function, pain, and health." *Am J Pain Manag* 4 (1994): 36–39.

Luckey, T D. "Radiation hormesis: the good, the bad, and the ugly.." *Dose-response : a publication of International Hormesis Society* 4.3 (2006): 169–190.

Mansi, Ishak et al. "Statins and musculoskeletal conditions, arthropathies, and injuries.." *JAMA internal medicine* 173.14 (2013): 1–10.

Mansi, Ishak et al. "Statins and New-Onset Diabetes Mellitus and Diabetic Complications: A Retrospective Cohort Study of US Healthy Adults.." *Journal of general internal medicine* 30.11 (2015): 1599–1610.

McDougall, Jean A et al. "Long-term statin use and risk of ductal and lobular breast cancer among women 55 to 74 years of age.." *Cancer epidemiology, biomarkers & prevention : a publication of the American Association for Cancer Research, cosponsored by the American Society of Preventive Oncology* 22.9 (2013): 1529–1537.

McGrath, Monica Forero, Mercedes L Kuroski de Bold, and Adolfo J de Bold. "The endocrine function of the heart.." *Trends in endocrinology and metabolism: TEM* 16.10 (2005): 469–477.

Meier-Ewert, Hans K et al. "Effect of sleep loss on C-reactive protein, an inflammatory marker of cardiovascular risk.." *Journal of the American College of Cardiology* 43.4 (2004): 678–683.

Mikus, Catherine R et al. "Simvastatin impairs exercise training adaptations.." *Journal of the American College of Cardiology* 62.8 (2013): 709–714.

Miller, Gregory E, Nicolas Rohleder, and Steve W Cole. "Chronic interpersonal stress predicts activation of pro- and anti-inflammatory signaling pathways 6 months later.." *Psychosomatic medicine* 71.1 (2009): 57–62.

Moore, Thomas et al. *Adverse Drug Reactions in Children Under Age 18.* Institute for Safe Medical Practices, June 12, 2014.

Morgan, Graeme, Robyn Ward, and Michael Barton. "The contribution of cytotoxic chemotherapy to 5-year survival in adult malignancies.." *Clinical oncology (Royal College of Radiologists (Great Britain))* 16.8 (2004): 549–560.

Morrison, D A, and J Sacks. "Balancing benefit against risk in the choice of therapy for coronary artery disease. Lesson from prospective, randomized, clinical trials of percutaneous coronary intervention and coronary artery bypass graft surgery.." *Minerva cardioangiologica* 51.5 (2003): 585–597.

Mozaffarian, Dariush et al. "Physical activity and incidence of atrial fibrillation in older adults: the cardiovascular health study.." *Circulation* 118.8 (2008): 800–807.

Nair, Shwetha et al. "Do slumped and upright postures affect stress responses? A randomized trial.." *Health psychology : official journal of the Division of Health Psychology, American Psychological Association* 34.6 (2015): 632–641.

Nave, Christopher S et al. "On the Contextual Independence of Personality: Teachers' Assessments Predict Directly Observed Behavior after Four Decades." *Social psychological and personality science* 3.1 (2010): 1–9.

Nichols, Jeanne F, Jacob E Palmer, and Susan S Levy. "Low bone mineral density in highly trained male master cyclists.." *Osteoporosis international : a journal established as result of cooperation between the European Foundation for Osteoporosis and the National Osteoporosis Foundation of the USA* 14.8 (2003): 644–649.

Null, Gary. *Death by medicine*. Mount Jackson, VA: Praktikos Books, 2011.

O'keefe, James H. "Organic Fitness: Achieving Hunter Gatherer Fitness in the 21 st Century." In, 2011.

Ogura, Takeshi et al. "Cerebral metabolic changes in men after chiropractic spinal manipulation for neck pain.." *Alternative Therapies in Health & Medicine* 17.6 (2011): 12–17.

Ornish, Dean. "Changing Your Lifestyle Can Change Your Genes." *Newsweek*, 16 Jun. 2008.

Ornish, Dean et al. "Changes in prostate gene expression in men undergoing an intensive nutrition and lifestyle intervention.." *Proceedings of the National Academy of Sciences of the United States of America* 105.24 (2008): 8369–8374.

Paddock, Catherine. "Danish Night Shift Workers Get Compensation For Cancer." *Medical News Today*, 17 Mar. 2009. Available: http://www.medicalnewstoday.com/articles/142454.php.

Pantell, Matthew et al. "Social Isolation: A Predictor of Mortality Comparable to Traditional Clinical Risk Factors." *American Journal of Public Health* 103.11 (2013): 2056–2062.

Park, Bum Jin et al. "The physiological effects of Shinrin-yoku (taking in the forest atmosphere or forest bathing): evidence from field experiments in 24 forests across Japan.." *Environmental health and preventive medicine* 15.1 (2010): 18–26.

Pettorossi, Vito Enrico, and Marco Schieppati. "Neck proprioception shapes body orientation and perception of motion." *Frontiers in human neuroscience* 8 (2014).

Pistolese, Richard A. "The Webster Technique: a chiropractic technique with obstetric implications.." *Journal of Manipulative and Physiological Therapeutics* 25.6 (2002): E1–9.

Polonsky, Kenneth S. "The Past 200 Years in Diabetes." *New England Journal of Medicine* 367.14 (2012): 1332–1340. Available: http://www.nejm.org/doi/full/10.1056/NEJMra1110560.

Prochazka, Allan V et al. "General health checks in adults for reducing morbidity and mortality from disease: summary review of primary findings and conclusions.." *JAMA internal medicine* 173.5 (2013): 371–372.

Ratey, J J, and E Hagerman, eds. *Spark! How exercise will improve the performance of your brain.* Quercus, 2008.

Rippe, James M, Theodore J Angelopoulos, and William F Rippe. "Lifestyle Medicine and Health Care Reform." *American Journal of Lifestyle Medicine* 3.6 (2009): 421–424. Available: http://orlandohealth.com/MediaBank/Docs/lifestyle_med/AJLM_Editorial_12-09.pdf.

Ripple, W J et al. "Status and ecological effects of the world's largest carnivores." *Science* (2014).

Roffers, S D, J M Menke, and D H Morris. "A Somatovisceral Reflex of Lowered Blood Pressure and Pulse Rate." *Asian Journal of Multidisciplinary ...* (2015).

Sahlins, Marshall. "The Original Affluent Society." *eco-action.org*, n.d. Online. Internet. 16 Nov. 2015. Available: http://www.eco-action.org/dt/affluent.html.

Sapolsky, R. *Why Zebras Don't Get Ulcers: A Guide to Stress, Stress Realted Diseases and Coping.* New York: W. H. Freeman, 1994.

Sarnat, Richard L, James Winterstein, and Jerrilyn A Cambron. "Clinical utilization and cost outcomes from an integrative medicine independent physician association: an additional 3-year update.." *Journal of Manipulative and Physiological Therapeutics* 30.4 (2007): 263–269.

Schulkin, Jay. *Allostasis, Homeostasis, and the Costs of Physiological Adaptation.* Cambridge University Press, 2004.

Schwartz, J G et al. *Does longterm endurance running enhance or inhibit coronary artery plaque formation? A prospective multidetector CTA study of men completing marathons for at least 25 consecutive years.* Journal of the American College of Cardiology, 2010.

Schwingshackl, Lukas, and Georg Hoffmann. "Dietary fatty acids in the secondary prevention of coronary heart disease: a systematic review, meta-analysis and meta-regression.." *BMJ open* 4.4 (2014): e004487.

Sharma, Tarang et al. "Suicidality and aggression during antidepressant treatment: systematic review and meta-analyses based on clinical study reports." *BMJ* (2016): i65.

Siri-Tarino, Patty W et al. "Meta-analysis of prospective cohort studies evaluating the association of saturated fat with cardiovascular disease." *The American Journal of Clinical Nutrition* (2010).

Spiegel, K, R Leproult, and E Van Cauter. "[Impact of sleep debt on physiological rhythms].." *Revue neurologique* 159.11 Suppl (2003): 6S11–20.

Suhrcke, Marc et al. *Chronic disease : an economic perspective.* London: Oxford Health Alliance, 2006.

Taleb, Naseem. *Antifragile: Things That Gain From Disorder.* New York: Random House, 2012.

van Leeuwen, Wessel M A et al. "Sleep restriction increases the risk of developing cardiovascular diseases by augmenting proinflammatory responses through IL-17 and CRP.." *PloS one* 4.2 (2009): e4589.

Vernacchio, L et al. "Medication use among children." *Pediatrics* 124.2 (2009).

Vincent, C, G Neale, and M Woloshynowych. "Adverse events in British hospitals: preliminary retrospective record review." *BMJ* 322.7285 (2001): 517–519.

Wannamethee, S Goya. "Height Loss in Older Men." *Archives of Internal Medicine* 166.22 (2006): 2546.

Waterland, R A, and R L Jirtle. "Transposable Elements: Targets for Early Nutritional Effects on Epigenetic Gene Regulation." *Molecular and Cellular Biology* 23.15 (2003): 5293–5300.

Weiss, Ram, Andrew A Bremer, and Robert H Lustig. "What is metabolic syndrome, and why are children getting it?." *Annals of the New York Academy of Sciences* 1281 (2013): 123–140.

West, K M. "Diabetes in American Indians and other native populations of the New World.." *Diabetes* 23.10 (1974): 841–855.

Winett, R A, and R N Carpinelli. "Potential health-related benefits of resistance training.." *Preventive medicine* 33.5 (2001): 503–513.

Wright, Kenneth P Jr et al. "Entrainment of the human circadian clock to the natural light-dark cycle.." *Current biology : CB* 23.16 (2013): 1554–1558.

Xie, Lulu et al. "Sleep drives metabolite clearance from the adult brain.." *Science* 342.6156 (2013): 373–377.

Zhang, John et al. "Effect of chiropractic care on heart rate variability and pain in a multisite clinical study.." *Journal of Manipulative and Physiological Therapeutics* 29.4 (2006): 267–274.

Across The Generations. Environmental Working Group, May 10, 2006. Available: http://www.ewg.org/research/across-generations/findings.

"Body Burden," 14 Jul. 2005. Online. Internet. 28 Apr. 2015. Available: http://www.ewg.org/research/body-burden-pollution-newborns.

Sitting Habits of Australian Workforce. Chiropractors' Association of Australia, January 1, 2012.

"Supernormal stimulus." *en.wikipedia.org*, n.d. Online. Internet. 17 Jan. 2016. Available: https://en.wikipedia.org/wiki/Supernormal_stimulus.

Teen girls' body burden of hormone-altering cosmetics chemicals: detailed findings. Environmental Working Group, September 24, 2008. Available: http://www.ewg.org/research/teen-girls-body-burden-hormone-altering-cosmetics-chemicals/detailed-findings.

"The economic and social costs of mental health problems in 2009/10." *Centre For Mental Health* (2010): 1–4. Available: http://www.centreformentalhealth.org.uk/news/2003_mental_illness_costs_over_77_billion.aspx.

"The Human Genome and Disappointment." *cbsnews.com*, n.d. Online. Internet. 25 Nov. 2015. Available: http://www.cbsnews.com/videos/extra-the-human-genome-disappointment/.

ENDNOTES

CHAPTER 2

D E Bloom, E T Cafiero, E Jan e Llopis, S Abrahams-Gessel, L R Bloom, S Fathima, A B Feigl, T Gaziano, M Mowafi, A Pandya, K Prettner, L Rosenberg, B Seligman, A Z Stein, and C Weinstein, "The Global Economic Burden of Non-communicable Diseases" *World Economic Forum.* (2012): 1–48.

James M Rippe, Theodore J Angelopoulos, and William F Rippe, "Lifestyle Medicine and Health Care Reform" *American Journal of Lifestyle Medicine.* 3.6 (2009): 421–424, Available: http://orlandohealth.com/MediaBank/Docs/lifestyle_med/AJLM_Editorial_12-09.pdf.

Marc Suhrcke et al., *Chronic disease : an economic perspective* (London: Oxford Health Alliance, 2006).

Bloom, Cafiero, Jan e Llopis, Abrahams-Gessel, Bloom, Fathima, Feigl, Gaziano, Mowafi, Pandya, Prettner, Rosenberg, Seligman, Stein, and Weinstein, "The Global Economic Burden of Non-communicable Diseases."

"The economic and social costs of mental health problems in 2009/10" *Centre For Mental Health.* (2010): 1–4, Available: http://www.centreformentalhealth.org.uk/news/2003_mental_illness_costs_over_77_billion.aspx.

Melonie Heron, "Deaths: leading causes for 2008." *National Vital Statistics Report.* 60.6 (2012): 1–94.

L Vernacchio et al., "Medication use among children" *Pediatrics.* 124.2 (2009).

C Vincent, G Neale, and M Woloshynowych, "Adverse events in British hospitals: preliminary retrospective record review" *BMJ.* 322.7285 (2001): 517–519.

T Jackson and A Harper, "Blunders will never cease. How the media report medical errors. A risky business" *BMJ.* 322.7285 (2001): 562.

Gary Null, *Death by medicine* (Mount Jackson, VA: Praktikos Books, 2011).

Phillip Aspden, ed., *Preventing Medical Errors* (Washinton DC: Institute of Medicine: Committee on Identifying and Preventing Medication Errors, 2007).

Charles M Kilo and Eric B Larson, "Exploring the harmful effects of health care." *JAMA.* 302.1 (2009): 89–91.

Allan V Prochazka et al., "General health checks in adults for reducing morbidity and mortality from disease: summary review of primary findings and conclusions." *JAMA internal medicine.* 173.5 (2013): 371–372.

William E Boden et al., "Impact of Optimal Medical Therapy With or Without Percutaneous Coronary Intervention on Lont-Term Cardiovascular End Points in Patients With Stable Coronary Artery Disease (from the Courage Trial" *The American Journal of Cardiology.* 104.1 (2009): 1–4.

D A Morrison and J Sacks, "Balancing benefit against risk in the choice of therapy for coronary artery disease. Lesson from prospective, randomized, clinical trials of percutaneous coronary intervention and coronary artery bypass graft surgery." *Minerva cardioangiologica.* 51.5 (2003): 585–597.

Action to Control Cardiovascular Risk in Diabetes Study Group et al., "Effects of intensive glucose lowering in type 2 diabetes." *New England Journal of Medicine.* 358.24 (2008): 2545–2559.

Kenneth S Polonsky, "The Past 200 Years in Diabetes" *New England Journal of Medicine.* 367.14 (2012): 1332–1340, Available: http://www.nejm.org/doi/full/10.1056/NEJMra1110560.

Graeme Morgan, Robyn Ward, and Michael Barton, "The contribution of cytotoxic chemotherapy to 5-year survival in adult malignancies." *Clinical oncology (Royal College of Radiologists (Great Britain)).* 16.8 (2004): 549–560.

Kilo and Larson, "Exploring the harmful effects of health care.."

Fitness Industry Association Great Britain, "Winning the Retention Battle: Reviewing Key Issues of UK Health & Fitness Club Membership Retention" (2001).

Prochazka et al., "General health checks in adults for reducing morbidity and mortality from disease: summary review of primary findings and conclusions.."

Jay Schulkin, *Allostasis, Homeostasis, and the Costs of Physiological Adaptation* (Cambridge University Press, 2004).

"The Human Genome and Disappointment" *cbsnews.com.* n.d., online, Internet, 25 Nov. 2015. Available: http://www.cbsnews.com/videos/extra-the-human-genome-disappointment/.

CHAPTER 3

Boden et al., "Impact of Optimal Medical Therapy With or Without Percutaneous Coronoary Intervention on Lont-Term Cardiovascular End Points in Patients With Stable Coronary Artery Disease (from the Courage Trial."

Morrison and Sacks, "Balancing benefit against risk in the choice of therapy for coronary artery disease. Lesson from prospective, randomized, clinical trials of percutaneous coronary intervention and coronary artery bypass graft surgery.."

Monica Forero McGrath, Mercedes L Kuroski de Bold, and Adolfo J de Bold, "The endocrine function of the heart." *Trends in endocrinology and metabolism: TEM.* 16.10 (2005): 469–477.

Catherine R Mikus et al., "Simvastatin impairs exercise training adaptations." *Journal of the American College of Cardiology.* 62.8 (2013): 709–714.

Ishak Mansi et al., "Statins and musculoskeletal conditions, arthropathies, and injuries." *JAMA internal medicine.* 173.14 (2013): 1–10.

Ishak Mansi et al., "Statins and New-Onset Diabetes Mellitus and Diabetic Complications: A Retrospective Cohort Study of US Healthy Adults." *Journal of general internal medicine.* 30.11 (2015): 1599–1610.

Jean A McDougall et al., "Long-term statin use and risk of ductal and lobular breast cancer among women 55 to 74 years of age." *Cancer epidemiology, biomarkers & prevention : a publication of the American Association for Cancer Research, cosponsored by the American Society of Preventive Oncology.* 22.9 (2013): 1529–1537.

Action to Control Cardiovascular Risk in Diabetes Study Group et al., "Effects of intensive glucose lowering in type 2 diabetes.."

Irving Kirsch, "Antidepressants and the Placebo Effect" *Zeitschrift für Psychologie.* 222.3 (2014): 128–134.

Tarang Sharma et al., "Suicidality and aggression during antidepressant treatment: systematic review and meta-analyses based on clinical study reports" *BMJ.* (2016): i65.

Naseem Taleb, *Antifragile: Things That Gain From Disorder* (New York: Random House, 2012).

Gerard Karsenty, "The complexities of skeletal biology." *Nature.* 423.6937 (2003): 316–318.

R A Waterland and R L Jirtle, "Transposable Elements: Targets for Early Nutritional Effects on Epigenetic Gene Regulation" *Molecular and Cellular Biology.* 23.15 (2003): 5293–5300.

A Ahlbom et al., "Cancer in twins: genetic and nongenetic familial risk factors." *Journal of the National Cancer Institute.* 89.4 (1997): 287–293.

David Dobbs, "The Social Life of Genes" *psmag.com.* n.d., online, Internet, 18 Nov. 2015. Available: http://www.psmag.com/books-and-culture/the-social-life-of-genes-64616.

James H O'keefe, "Organic Fitness: Achieving Hunter Gatherer Fitness in the 21 st Century"in. 2011.

Dean Ornish, "Changing Your Lifestyle Can Change Your Genes" *Newsweek.* 16 Jun. 2008.

Dean Ornish et al., "Changes in prostate gene expression in men undergoing an intensive nutrition and lifestyle intervention." *Proceedings of the National Academy of Sciences of the United States of America*. 105.24 (2008): 8369–8374.

Jorge Alejandro Alegria-Torres, Andrea Baccarelli, and Valentina Bollati, "Epigenetics and lifestyle." *Epigenomics*. 3.3 (2011): 267–277.

W J Ripple et al., "Status and ecological effects of the world's largest carnivores" *Science*. (2014).

T D Luckey, "Radiation hormesis: the good, the bad, and the ugly." *Dose-response: a publication of International Hormesis Society*. 4.3 (2006): 169–190.

CHAPTER 5

R Sapolsky, *Why Zebras Don't Get Ulcers: A Guide to Stress, Stress Realted Diseases and Coping* (New York: W. H. Freeman, 1994).

Schulkin, *Allostasis, Homeostasis, and the Costs of Physiological Adaptation*.

M Gurven and H Kaplan, "Longevity among hunter-gatherers: a cross-cultural examination" *Population and Development Review*. (2007).

H O Lancaster, *Expectations of Life: A Study in the Demography, Statistics, and History of World Mortality* Springer Science & Business Media. (1990).

K M West, *Diabetes in American Indians and other native populations of the New World*. Diabetes. 23.10 (1974): 841–855.

Body Burden Environmental Working Group 14 Jul. 2005, Available: http://www.ewg.org/research/body-burden-pollution-newborns.

Teen girls' body burden of hormone-altering cosmetic chemicals: detailed findings Environmental Working Group, September 24, 2008, Available: http://www.ewg.org/research/teen-girls-body-burden-hormone-altering-cosmetics-chemicals/detailed-findings.

Across The Generations Environmental Working Group, May 10, 2006, Available: http://www.ewg.org/research/across-generations/findings.

CHAPTER 6

Goran Bjelakovic et al., "Mortality in Randomized Trials of Antioxidant Supplements for Primary and Secondary Prevention" *JAMA*. 297.8 (2007): 842.

Ram Weiss, Andrew A Bremer, and Robert H Lustig, "What is metabolic syndrome, and why are children getting it?" *Annals of the New York Academy of Sciences*. 1281 (2013): 123–140.

CHAPTER 6

Goran Bjelakovic et al., "Mortality in Randomized Trials of Antioxidant Supplements for Primary and Secondary Prevention" *JAMA*. 297.8 (2007): 842.

Ram Weiss, Andrew A Bremer, and Robert H Lustig, "What is metabolic syndrome, and why are children getting it?" *Annals of the New York Academy of Sciences*. 1281 (2013): 123–140.

CHAPTER 7

P Brickman et al., "Lottery winners and accident victims: is happiness relative?" *Journal of personality and social psychology*. 36.8 (1978): 917–927.

CHAPTER 8

Marshall Sahlins, "The Original Affluent Society" *eco-action.org*. n.d., online, Internet, 16 Nov. 2015. Available: http://www.eco-action.org/dt/affluent.html.

"Supernormal stimulus" *en.wikipedia.org*. n.d., online, Internet, 17 Jan. 2016. Available: https://en.wikipedia.org/wiki/Supernormal_stimulus.

F Forencich, *Change Your Body, Change The World* (Exuberant Animal Books, 2010).

CHAPTER 9

Heidi Haavik and Bernadette Murphy, "Subclinical Neck Pain and the Effects of Cervical Manipulation on Elbow Joint Position Sense" *Journal of Manipulative and Physiological Therapeutics*. 34.2 (2011): 88–97.

E R Kandel et al., *Principles of Neural Science*, vol., Fifth Edition. (McGraw-Hill, 2012).

John Zhang et al., "Effect of chiropractic care on heart rate variability and pain in a multisite clinical study." *Journal of Manipulative and Physiological Therapeutics*. 29.4 (2006): 267–274.

Takeshi Ogura et al., "Cerebral metabolic changes in men after chiropractic spinal manipulation for neck pain." *Alternative Therapies in Health & Medicine*. 17.6 (2011): 12–17.

Heidi Haavik and Bernadette Murphy, "The role of spinal manipulation in addressing disordered sensorimotor integration and altered motor control." *Journal of electromyography and kinesiology : official journal of the International Society of Electrophysiological Kinesiology*. 22.5 (2012): 768–776.

S D Roffers, J M Menke, and D H Morris, "A Somatovisceral Reflex of Lowered Blood Pressure and Pulse Rate" *Asian Journal of Multidisciplinary* .... (2015).

G Bakris et al., "Atlas vertebra realignment and achievement of arterial pressure goal in hypertensive patients: a pilot study." *Journal of human hypertension.* 21.5 (2007): 347–352.

Richard L Sarnat, James Winterstein, and Jerrilyn A Cambron, "Clinical utilization and cost outcomes from an integrative medicine independent physician association: an additional 3-year update." *Journal of Manipulative and Physiological Therapeutics.* 30.4 (2007): 263–269.

Joan Fallon, "The effect of chiropractic treatment on pregnancy and labor: a comprehensive study" *Proceedings of the World Federation of Chiropractic.* (1991): 24–31.

Richard A Pistolese, "The Webster Technique: a chiropractic technique with obstetric implications." *Journal of Manipulative and Physiological Therapeutics.* 25.6 (2002): E1–9.

M S Gottlieb, "Neglected spinal cord, brain stem and musculoskeletal injuries stemming from birth trauma." *Journal of Manipulative and Physiological Therapeutics.* 16.8 (1993): 537–543.

J Barham-Floreani and S Floreani, *The Legitimacy of Chiropractic in Family Healthcare* (Well Adjusted, September 3, 2013).

Matthew F Doyle, "Is chiropractic paediatric care safe? A best evidence topic" *Clinical Chiropractic.* 14.3 (n.d.): 97–105.

Thomas Moore et al., *Adverse Drug Reactions in Children Under Age 18* (Institute for Safe Medical Practices, June 12, 2014).

John Lennon et al., "Postural and respiratory modulation of autonomic function, pain, and health" *Am J Pain Manag.* 4 (1994): 36–39.

René Cailliet and Leonard Gross, "The rejuvenation strategy" (1988); Ian J Edwards, Susan A Deuchars, and Jim Deuchars, "The intermedius nucleus of the medulla: a potential site for the integration of cervical information and the generation of autonomic responses" *Journal of chemical neuroanatomy.* 38.3 (2009): 166–175; Vito Enrico Pettorossi and Marco Schieppati, "Neck proprioception shapes body orientation and perception of motion" *Frontiers in human neuroscience.* 8 (2014).

Deborah M Kado et al., "Hyperkyphotic Posture and Poor Physical Functional Ability in Older Community-Dwelling Men and Women: The Rancho Bernardo Study" *The journals of gerontology. Series A, Biological sciences and medical sciences.* 60.5 (2005): 633–637.

S Goya Wannamethee, "Height Loss in Older Men" *Archives of Internal Medicine.* 166.22 (2006): 2546.

Dana R Carney, Amy J C Cuddy, and Andy J Yap, "Power Posing: Brief Nonverbal Displays Affect Neuroendocrine Levels and Risk Tolerance" *Psychological Science.* 21.10 (2010): 1363–1368.

Shwetha Nair et al., "Do slumped and upright postures affect stress responses? A randomized trial." *Health psychology : official journal of the Division of Health Psychology, American Psychological Association.* 34.6 (2015): 632–641.

A Breig, *Biomechanics of the Nervous System: Breig revisited*, Ed. M Shacklock, vol., First. (Adelaide: Neurodynamic Solutions, 2007).

CHAPTER 10

E Chen et al., "Genome-wide transcriptional profiling linked to social class in asthma" *Thorax.* 64.1 (2009): 38–43.

Christopher S Nave et al., "On the Contextual Independence of Personality: Teachers' Assessments Predict Directly Observed Behavior after Four Decades" *Social psychological and personality science.* 3.1 (2010): 1–9.

Matthew Pantell et al., "Social Isolation: A Predictor of Mortality Comparable to Traditional Clinical Risk Factors" *American Journal of Public Health.* 103.11 (2013): 2056–2062.

DOBBS, "The Social Life of Genes."

S W Cole, M E Kemeny, and S E Taylor, "Social identity and physical health: accelerated HIV progression in rejection-sensitive gay men." *Journal of personality and social psychology.* 72.2 (1997): 320–335; S W Cole et al., "Accelerated course of human immunodeficiency virus infection in gay men who conceal their homosexual identity." *Psychosomatic medicine.* 58.3 (1996): 219–231; S W Cole et al., "Elevated physical health risk among gay men who conceal their homosexual identity." *Health psychology : official journal of the Division of Health Psychology, American Psychological Association.* 15.4 (1996): 243–251.

Gregory E Miller, Nicolas Rohleder, and Steve W Cole, "Chronic interpersonal stress predicts activation of pro- and anti-inflammatory signaling pathways 6 months later." *Psychosomatic medicine.* 71.1 (2009): 57–62.

Joan Kaufman et al., "Social supports and serotonin transporter gene moderate depression in maltreated children." *Proceedings of the National Academy of Sciences of the United States of America.* 101.49 (2004): 17316–17321.